1001 little
HEALTH
MIRACLES

Simple solutions that
provide big benefits

Esme Floyd

CARLTON
BOOKS

THIS IS A CARLTON BOOK

Text and design copyright © 2004
Carlton Books Limited

This edition published in 2011 by
Carlton Books Limited
20 Mortimer Street
London W1T 3JW

ISBN 978 1 84732 945 5

Printed and bound in China

Senior Executive Editor: Lisa Dyer
Art Director: Lucy Coley
Design: Penny Stock
Copy Editors: Libby Willis and Jonathan Hilton
Illustrator: Kerrie Hess
Production: Rachel Burgess

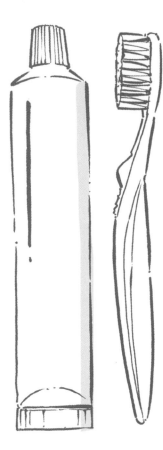

1001 little
HEALTH
MIRACLES

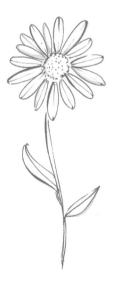

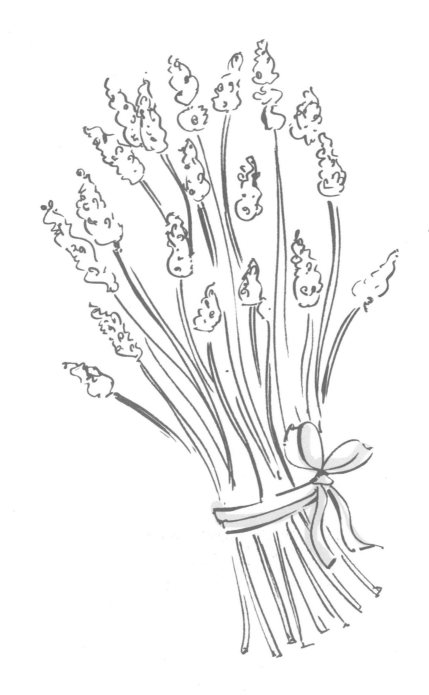

CONTENTS

INTRODUCTION

Did you know that wrapping presents could help you burn 100 calories an hour, or that butter could actually be better for you than low-fat alternatives?

Here we've gathered together 1001 little health gems, based on current scientific evidence, to help you stay happy and healthy in every area of your life. Simply read through the book or dip in and out according to how you feel. From hayfever cures to workout wisdom, from travel problems to beating stress, the book contains advice to help make your life brighter and better.

Top ten little health miracles

80
EAT APPLES TO FIGHT THE BULGE
(see Fighting fat, page 25)

107
EASE PAIN WITH CHERRIES
(see Miracle foods, page 31)

221
HAVE A BRAZILIAN
(see Energy-boosters, page 56)

DIET & NUTRITION

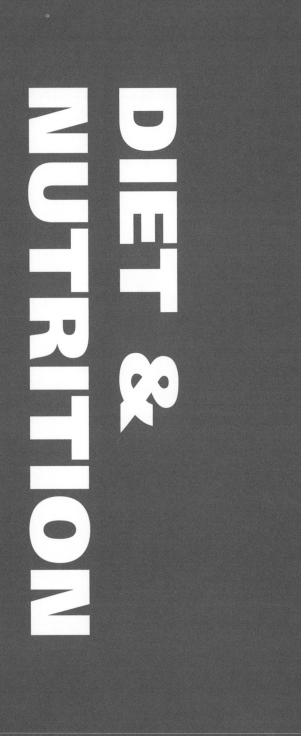

alcohol

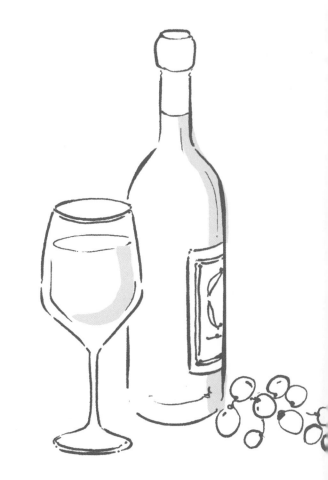

1 DON'T GIVE UP

Alcohol increases your levels of HDL, the healthier form of cholesterol. It also decreases the chances of clogged arteries, so a reasonable amount of alcohol in the diet could be more beneficial than abstinence.

2 AVOID FLUSHING AWAY FOLATE

Alcohol reduces folic acid and vitamin B6, both of which are essential for the body to protect against a range of diseases and conditions, including breast cancer. If you drink regularly, make sure you're getting enough folic acid (found in liver, fortified breakfast cereals, leafy green vegetables and numerous supplements).

3 CUT DOWN TO CUT THE CALORIES

Every gram of alcohol contains around 7 calories, so if your aim is to lose weight, remember how quickly those little tipples could topple the scales.

4 TWO'S THE LIMIT FOR HEALTHY BREASTS

Women who have three or more drinks a day are nearly a third more likely to develop breast cancer compared with women who don't drink alcohol, so to protect your breasts choose a non-alcoholic drink or stick to just one or two glasses a day.

5 DRINK YOURSELF PINK

Drinking just one or two glasses of wine a day could cut your risk of heart disease by up to a third, and red and rosé wines may be even more beneficial than white wine because of the higher levels of antioxidants they contain.

6 KEEP IN THE CLEAR

Spirits and dark alcoholic drinks contain higher levels of substances called congeners, which can be toxic to the brain and nervous system. This is why, if you drink whisky, you're more likely to have a hangover the next day than if you drink white wine. Stick to clear drinks for a clear head.

7 BEWARE OF A BEER BELLY

Experts believe that just two pints of beer (40fl oz) a day can counter the beneficial effects on the colon of a healthy diet full of fresh fruit and vegetables, increasing suseptibility to colon cancer by reducing folic acid levels.

8 UNDER 21S ONLY

Keeping your alcohol consumption in the low-to-moderate band has proven benefits for your health. Women who drink more than 21 units of alcohol a week could be endangering their heart – drinking heavily could increase their risk of coronary heart disease by 57%.

9 GO INTO THE RED

Red wine contains a health-boosting flavonoid called reservatrol, which is a natural chemical found in grape skins. This substance may prevent a range of health problems, including heart disease, strokes, brain diseases and even some cancers.

10 TAKE HEART WITH A BOTTLE OF BEER

Beer provides one important nutrient group – the B vitamins. Half a pint (10fl oz) of beer provides 17% of the recommended daily amount (RDA) of the important B vitamin folic acid, which has been linked to lowering the risk of heart disease.

11 NESTLE DOWN WITH A NIGHTCAP

Just 1 unit (drink) of alcohol (half a pint of beer, a small glass of wine, one standard measure of spirits) can produce a relaxing effect to help you sleep – once in a while.

calories

12 GO NUTTY FOR WEIGHT LOSS

Nuts might be high in calories, but thanks to the construction of their cell walls, our body can't access them all, which means they're even healthier than once thought. Almonds are particularly nutritious.

13 CLEAN UP TO BURN UP

Cleaning and general housework around the home, such as mopping the floor or vacuuming the carpet, burns off an incredible 233 calories an hour, which is the equivalent of a bagel.

14 GO THE EXTRA MILE

Experts suggest that to lose weight you need to eliminate 500 calories a day. For most people, this means an hour of walking at a rate of 12 minutes per mile.

15 THINK TWICE BEFORE YOU GRAB THAT BURGER

To use up the calories you'd get from an average fast-food burger, you'd need to cycle for at least 90 minutes.
Choose low-calorie alternatives such as ciabatta, wholegrain sandwiches or pasta instead.

16 GO SKINNY TO SKIM OFF CALORIES

Choosing a coffee with skimmed milk rather than whole milk could save you the same amount of calories as 20 minutes of moderate cycling.

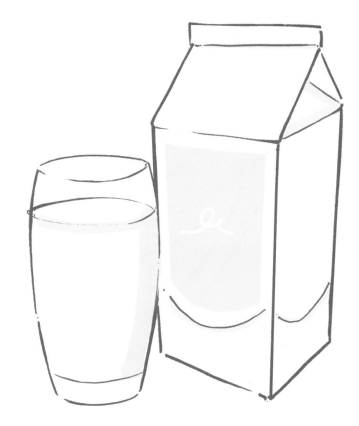

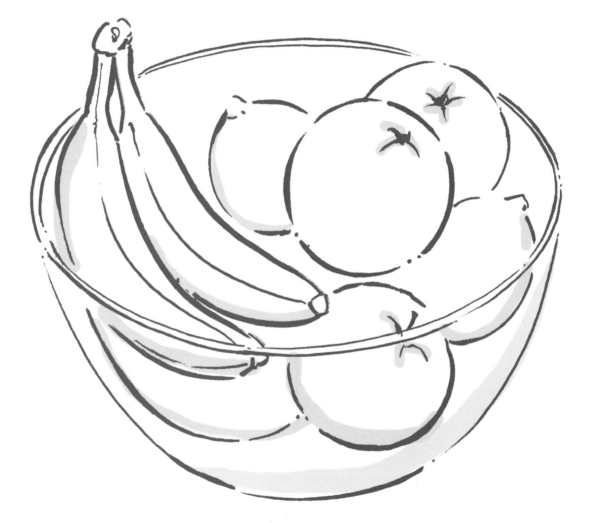

17 FILL UP ON FRUIT

Fruit contains fructose so it has more calories than salad or vegetables, but an apple or orange will still give you only around 80 calories, as opposed to a whopping 600 for a cheeseburger.

18 SHAVE PORTIONS TO SHED INCHES

A great way to shave off calories without losing the taste of your food is to eat smaller portions. Reducing the size of a steak from 150g to 75g (5oz to 3oz) could save more than 200 calories.

19 CHEW THOSE CALORIES AWAY

Replacing a packet of full-sugar chewing gum with a sugar-free variety could save 100 calories.

20 FAVOUR LOW-FAT FILLINGS

Changing the mayonnaise in your sandwich from full fat to low fat could save the same amount of calories as you'd burn up doing an extra hour at work.

21 CHOOSE TO BE CHOOSY

A variety in food choices encourages over-eating because we tend to want to try different flavours and textures. Fight this natural urge by surrounding yourself with low-caloriebut high-flavour foods.

22 GET FULL WITH THE FIZZ

Swapping a sugary drink or glass of wine for sparkling water at lunchtime could save hundreds of calories over the week.

23 WRAP IT UP

Did you know you can use up 100 calories an hour wrapping presents? What a perfect excuse to buy gifts!

24 THINK THIN AND TALL

People perceive tall, thin glasses to hold more than short ones, and drink 20% more from stubbier ones. For high-calorie drinks, like fruit juice, smoothies or alcohol, use tall, narrow glasses. You'll think you drank more than you actually did.

25 TAKE YOUR TIME IN THE BATHROOM

Don't skimp on getting glam before you go out. Doing your hair and make-up helps you burn off a fantastic 166 calories an hour.

cholesterol

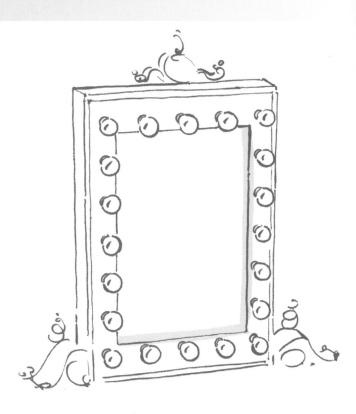

26 GET A GOOD BALANCE

Total blood cholesterol measures the amount of cholesterol circulating in the blood. The LDL level is a measure of damaging low-density lipoproteins, thought to be responsible for many health problems. HDL (high-density lipoproteins), or 'good' cholesterol, is thought to be much less damaging.

27 GET IN PEAK FORM WITH PECANS

Adding pecans to your diet not only lowers total cholesterol and levels of LDL, or 'bad' cholesterol, but can also help maintain HDL, or 'good' cholesterol, in the blood.

28 SEE RED TO REDUCE CHOLESTEROL

A Chinese rice preparation called Red Yeast Rice has been shown in recent studies to reduce cholesterol when used as a food supplement. This preparation works by soaking up damaging serum cholesterol and triglycerides contained in the blood.

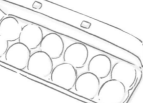

29 GET EGG-CELLENT RESULTS

Far from eggs being
the bad guys in the fight
against cholesterol in the bloodstream, it is now thought that certain
compounds found in eggs may actually
prevent the absorption of cholesterol into
the body if one a day is eaten.

30 HAVE A MINI-DRIVE

More frequent mini-meals or light snacks
that spread out your calorie intake evenly
throughout the entire day help maintain
a steady balance in blood chemistry,
avoiding peaks and dips in blood sugar
and lowering cholesterol.

31 BOOST GOOD CHOLESTEROL

Vegetables, fruit, fibre and wholegrains
boost levels of HDL in the bloodstream
when eaten regularly. Aim for one of
each of these foodstuffs at every meal.

32 GET CLUED UP ON GARLIC CLOVES

Garlic contains allicin, a cholesterol-fighting
substance that inhibits the retention of bad
LDL cholesterol in the blood vessels and
encourages its elimination from the body.

33 PRUNE BACK BLOOD CHOLESTEROL

Prunes contain high
levels of
antioxidants that
help lower stored
levels of damaging
LDL, making them
a perfect quick
snack.

34 DRINK TO FEEL SWELL

Drinking 2–3 litres (3½–5¼ pints)
of water a day helps fight cholesterol
because water encourages the fibre in food
to swell and stimulates the liver to produce
HDL, while lowering the rate at which
the body absorbs fat.

35 TEAM UP FAT AND FIBRE

The saturated animal fats contained in some foods encourage the liver to produce LDL, but the damaging effect of this substance is reduced if the food is accompanied by a source of fibre and some water. For instance, snack on cheese, wholegrain bread and a glass of water.

36 BE NUTS ABOUT HEALTHY BLOOD

Almonds, hazelnuts, macadamia nuts and oils such as rapeseed and olive contain high levels of monounsaturated fats, which help reduce cholesterol and restore the good–bad balance.

37 BUTTER YOURSELF BETTER

Butter has often been thought to be a cholesterol villain because of its high saturated fat levels, but butter alternatives like hydrogenated margarines and cooking fats (other than olive oil) could in fact be worse because of their high levels of trans fats, which lower HDL levels in the body.

38 BOTTOMS UP FOR BETTER BALANCE

One or two glasses of antioxidant-rich wine or beer a day will not only encourage your body to produce HDL – the anthocyanins and other antioxidants they contain can also lower LDL.

39 SWEAT HEALTH TROUBLES AWAY

Physical exercise is a factor in reducing the levels of destructive LDL in the bloodstream, thus restoring a good cholesterol balance and helping your system maintain health. For the best results, aim for between three and four workouts every week.

40 C AND E YOUR ARTERIES

Healthy arteries contract and expand an average of 70 times every minute to move blood around your body, undergoing enormous pressure swings as a result. Recent studies have shown that vitamins C and E can help the artery walls to stay elastic and strong.

41 FISHING FOR HEALTHY ARTERIES

Oily fish, including salmon, mackerel, sardines, herrings and fresh tuna, contain omega-3 essential fatty acids (EFAs) that prevent LDL from being deposited in the arteries and blood clots from forming.

42 GIVE YOUR LIVER A BREAK

Only about 20% of the cholesterol in the body is ingested directly through the diet. A whopping 80% is produced by the liver in response to processed foods and saturated fats. Eating fruits, vegetables, wholegrains and oily fish stops your liver having to work so hard.

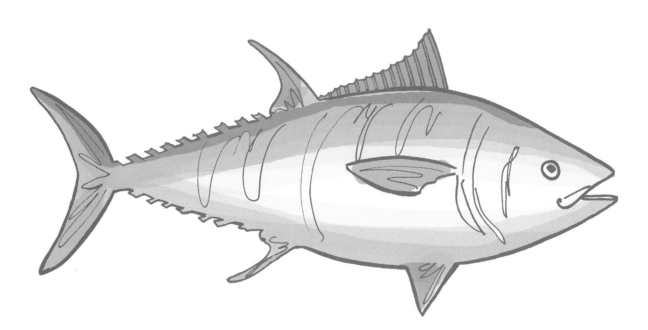

43 SHARE THE CHARDONNAY

It might sound an unlikely ally in the fight against cholesterol, but research has revealed that just a glass of Chardonnay a day might help your body get rid of damaging cholesterol.

44 JUICE AWAY BAD CHOLESTEROL

Drinking three small glasses of orange juice every day could not only reduce LDL levels in the blood but also boost levels of HDL by up to a fifth, making it a great choice for heart health.

dehydration

45 COUNT TO EIGHT

Water suppresses the appetite naturally and helps the body metabolize stored fat, actually reducing fat deposits. Make sure you get your eight glasses a day if you want to stay slim.

46 DRINK UP TO TONE UP

Drinking the right amount of water helps maintain muscle tone by giving muscles their natural ability to contract, so making sure you don't get dehydrated helps you tone up and strengthen up, too.

47 DON'T WAIT TILL YOU'RE THIRSTY

If you feel thirsty, you're already dehydrated. Aim to drink little and often throughout the day so you never get to the stage where you feel thirsty.

48 GULP DOWN A CLEAR WINNER

Alcohol and drinks that contain caffeine, especially coffee and colas, cause rather than protect against dehydration. Choose plain water instead.

49 DRINK TO FEEL DYNAMIC

Feelings of anxiety and confusion, and having dry skin, an increased heart rate, decreased blood pressure and even fainting can all be signs of dehydration.

50 GO RAW FOR GOOD FLUID RESERVES

You can supplement your fluid intake by
eating raw fruits and vegetables, such
as tomatoes, broccoli, lettuce, carrots,
watermelon, grapefruit and apples. All
of these fruits and vegetables contain high
levels of water.

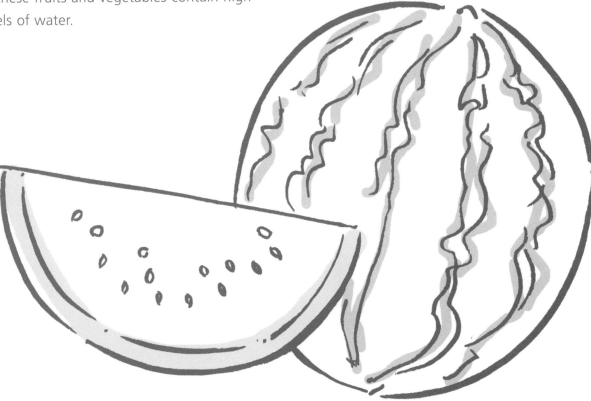

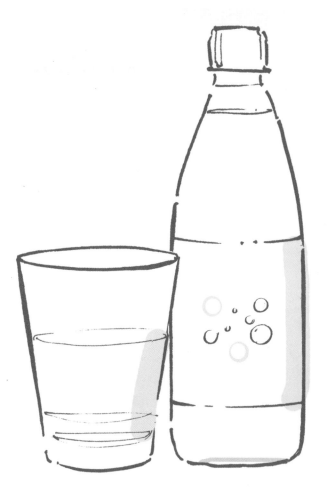

51 STAY SHARP WITH REGULAR SIPPING

A major effect of dehydration is on concentration. If you're dehydrated, you'll stop being able to think clearly and experts believe this is why many people have an afternoon lull. To keep alert, drink water throughout the day.

52 PROTECT MUSCLES WITH WATER

Water in the body binds to muscle glycogen at a rate of 4 grams to every gram of glycogen. If you starve your body of water or food, these groups are split up and although you might lose weight, it's not the right weight to lose.

53 DON'T WATER DOWN YOUR HEALTH

Water makes up between 50% and 70% of the human body and is the essential constituent of blood, lymph, digestive juices, urine and perspiration. Without it, your body simply can't function, and experts recommend you drink 1.5–2 litres (2½–3½ pints) spread throughout the day.

54 DON'T FORGET TO SWEAT

If you allow your body to become dehydrated during exercise, you lose the ability to sweat and cool off, which can raise body temperatures to dangerous levels – 80% of temperature regulation occurs through perspiration.

55 DAMP DOWN ON DEHYDRATION

When exercising in hot or humid conditions, you can lose 2–3 litres (3½–5¼ pints) of water per hour, leaving an average-sized woman dehydrated after only half an hour's activity. Drinking two glasses of water before you work out sets you up for a successful session.

56 CLEAR UP YOUR MEMORY

It might not sound much, but a mere 2% drop in your body's water levels – 1 litre (1¾ pints) of water for someone who weighs 68kg (10st 10lb/150lbs) – results in short-term memory impairment, trouble with basic maths and difficulty in focusing.

57 DROWN OUT CHOLESTEROL

When dehydrated, your body produces cholesterol, which surrounds the cells to protect the fluids within them. In the long term, this can damage general health.

58 SHIFT MORE WEIGHT BY DRINKING UP

Dehydration can slow down metabolism as it springs the body into starvation mode and holds onto fat cells that contain high levels of fluids. So drink up to keep your metabolism rate high.

59 FLUSH AWAY CANCER

Studies have shown that drinking at least five glasses of water a day can significantly decrease the risk of cancers of the colon, bladder and breast.

60 SAY AAHHH

Your tongue is a good indicator of general health. If it doesn't look pink and fleshy, you could be dehydrated or have a chronic health problem, such as sugar imbalance.

detox

61 GET ENERGETIC WITH A CLEANSING TONIC

Try this cleansing tonic to help strengthen your liver: 200ml (7fl oz) spring water, juice of a lemon, pinch of powdered ginger, 1 tablespoon flaxseeds, 1 teaspoon psyllium powder.

62 PRACTISE YOUR BRUSHSTROKE

Dry body brushing before showering has been shown to stimulate lymphatic flow and circulation and remove dead skin cells. You'll need a soft bristle brush with a long detachable handle, to enable you to reach right down your back.

63 DRESS IN LEMON AND GINGER

Avoid caffeine, alcohol, refined sugar and salt. Instead, season your food with lemon juice, garlic, ginger or cayenne pepper, all of which support the detox process while adding flavour.

64 GET A PEPPER PICK-UP

Chilli and cayenne pepper are excellent additions to a detox regime because they impart a whole lot of taste to food while helping the body eliminate toxins and cutting down on hunger pangs and food cravings.

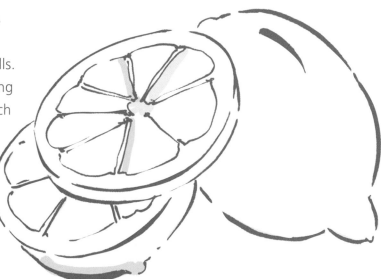

65 PURIFY WITH A HOME BREW

Make a purifying herb tea from 1 teaspoon each of nettle, peppermint, dandelion root and red clover combined in a saucepan with 3 cups of cold water. Bring to the boil, reduce the heat and simmer for 15 minutes. Strain and sweeten with apple juice if required.

66 SPLASH OUT WITH SALSA

Use hot tomato salsa as an alternative to butter or mayonnaise to add spicy flavour to your baked potatoes and as a piquant accompaniment to meat and fish. It tastes delicious and the chilli and tomatoes help your body detox.

67 FL-OAT TOXINS AWAY

Oats are a great food for detoxing as they help the body flush out toxins as well as releasing their energy slowly into the body to prevent cravings (unrolled oats are more effective at this) and lowering cholesterol in the blood.

fighting fat

68 GET HIP WITH HEMP

Use hemp oil as a low-fat alternative to butter and vegetable oils in cooking. Not only is it low in fat, it's also high in omega-3 and omega-6 essential fatty acids (EFAs).

68 KNOW YOUR NUMBERS

For every 10g of fat contained in a meal, women store nearly 4g in subcutaneous tissue (men store less than half this amount), so knowing how much fat is on your plate will help you work out how much exercise you will need to do to burn it off! The recommended daily fat intake for an average woman is 70g (2½oz).

70 LOSE A BITTER FAT

Bitter orange, aka *citrus aurantium*, stimulates weight loss by increasing the production of heat to burn fat calories at a faster rate, giving the body access to greater amounts of energy.

71 DROP THE DRESSING TO DROP A DRESS SIZE

The average woman gets more fat from salad dressing than from any other food source. Just 2 tablespoons of salad dressing can contain between 10g and 20g of fat. To lighten up, try oil-free dressings or choose fat-free lemon juice instead.

72 COUNT ON CHROMIUM

Chromium helps control sugar cravings and suppress appetite, but many people's diets don't contain very much of this element because the natural soil reserves fresh produce is grown in are slowly being depleted; a supplement may help.

73 LINK STEAK AND SPINACH TO STAY LEAN

The amino acid L-carnitine, contained in lean meat, helps the body burn fat and it works even better when it's combined with vegetables such as spinach that contain another amino acid called lysine.

74 GIVE FAT THE COLD SHOULDER

A good and simple way to help your body fight fat is to drink ice-cold water. This causes more calories to be used up by the body than drinking water at room temperature because the digestive system has to use extra energy to heat it to body temperature.

75 BURN FAT WHILE YOU REST

Exercising regularly helps boost your metabolism because muscle cells require more energy than fat cells in order to function. People who take regular exercise burn off about 600 more calories a week (and that is equivalent to the calories in four pieces of cheesecake!).

76 GET BREADY TO GET THINNER

Wholewheat bread, wheatgerm, brown rice and peanuts all contain high levels of thiamine (vitamin B1), which helps the body convert carbohydrates to energy and reduce fat deposits.

77 BE A FAT SLEUTH

Don't be seduced by the various 'low-fat' claims found on some food labels. 'Reduced fat' means the food has 25% less fat than the standard version, but it could still be a high-fat food and many contain refined sugar, which actually prompts weight gain.

78 FIX ON 45

If you are exercising at a steady pace, you need to keep going for more than 45 minutes before your body's potential for burning fat is optimal.

79 GO GREEN TO DROP WEIGHT

As well as containing metabolism-boosting caffeine, green tea has a secret ingredient with thermogenic properties. This means it increases energy production and stimulates fat oxidation in the body.

80 EAT APPLES TO FIGHT THE BULGE

The high levels of leptin in apples and celery help the body metabolize fat cells and reduce fat storage in subcutaneous layers, helping you stay smooth and slim.

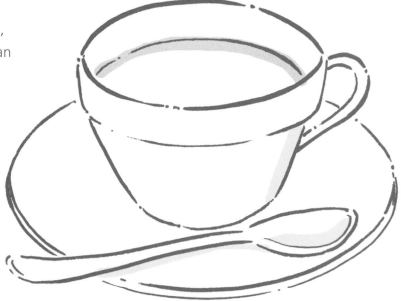

81 ATTACK FAT WITH BLADDERWRACK

Scientists are beginning to turn to plants in the fight against obesity and they have discovered that bladderwrack (*fuscus vesiculosus*) can stimulate the metabolism, aiding weight loss and successfully treating obesity.

82 ADD FLAVONOIDS TO BOOST METABOLISM

Fresh fruit and vegetables contain high levels of flavonoids, which not only act as antioxidants in the body but also boost basic metabolism, helping weight loss by altering enzymes involved in metabolism and cell growth.

83 A SEEDY WAY TO LOSE FAT

Eating some seeds instead of a high-fat snack could doubly boost weight loss by increasing your intake of leucine – found in soya, whey, nuts and seeds – which reduces body fat during weight loss.

84 BUILD MUSCLE TO BURN CALORIES AT REST

Muscle is the most metabolically active part of your body and burns up to three times as many calories as any other tissue. Add some resistance training to your workout to boost lean muscle and help you burn off calories in your downtime.

85 COMBINE FOOD GROUPS

Pyruvate, a substance created in the body as it digests and metabolizes carbohydrates and proteins, has been shown to promote weight loss, so beware of faddy diets that separate carbs and proteins.

86 KEEP A DIARY

Keeping a food diary is a good method of cutting down on your calorie intake by making yourself aware of how much you really eat every day, and what your weaknesses are. Then rebalance your diet in favour of low-fat fruits, vegetables and complex carbohydrates.

87 DON'T DRINK YOURSELF FAT

All alcohol is high in calories – bear in mind that drinking just three pints of beer (about four bottles of beer) could add up to 600 calories to your intake. Sugary drinks should also be limited. A can of cola contains 135 calories, and apart from the energy it has virtually no nutritional value.

88 BALANCE FAT AT 20%

Keeping fat calories to 20% of total calorie consumption is ideal. Make up the rest with fibre-rich wholegrain breads, brown rice, pulses (legumes), and fresh fruit and a variety of vegetables.

89 GET FAT LOSS DOWN TO A TEA

Caffeine interacts with the body's hormones to increase the rate at which calories are burned, and studies have shown that tea and green tea are more beneficial sources for the body than coffee.

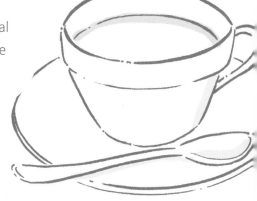

indulgences

90 FLAVOUR FOR HEART HEALTH

Artificial flavours may not all be bad news for health. Some contain salicylates, a chemical cousin of aspirin, which could actually help protect against circulation problems by thinning the blood.

91 INDULGE YOUR SWEET TOOTH FOR A LONGER LIFE

Chocolate may not only make your sweet tooth happy, it may also lengthen your life, possibly due to antioxidant chemicals present in chocolate, but also thanks to the mood boost that the indulgence gives you. Dark varieties with 70% cocoa are best.

92 GUILT-FREE CHOCOLATE TREATS

Chocolate is rich in antioxidants called phenols – substances that offer some protection against heart disease – while the fat in chocolate (stearic acid) is converted by the body into oleic acid, which is a monounsaturated fat found in olive oil.

93 FATTEN UP YOUR BONES

Women who eat more fat have higher calcium absorption rates than women on low-fat diets because fat slows down calcium's transit time through the intestines, thus increasing the opportunity for absorption.

94 INDULGE YOUR SCENT-SES

Most of the tastes we love are strongly determined by our sense of smell. So the next time you desire a treat, try inhaling its aroma deeply instead of putting the item straight in your mouth. Often, the smell can be satisfying enough.

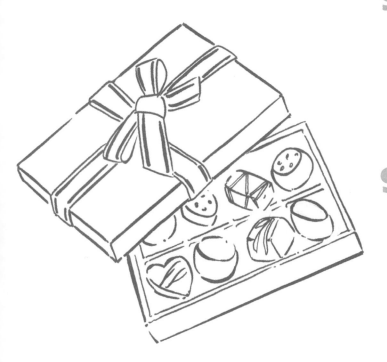

95 BEAT PMS WITH CHOCOLATE

Chocolate, far from being all bad, has been shown to ease the symptoms of PMS and depression, as well as containing phenols, a type of antioxidant that is thought to protect the health of the heart as well as lower cholesterol.

96 SAY CHEESE FOR A WHITER SMILE

The calcium and phosphate found in cheese combine with saliva in the mouth to prevent erosion of the top layer of enamel on the teeth. As an added benefit, the high percentage of fat in cheese helps calcium absorption in the body.

97 FEEL FULLER WITH NUTS

Recent research has found that eating a handful of peanuts every day can help you reduce your weight. This is because the peanuts produce a feeling of fullness, which, in turn, means you eat less later. The nuts also lower fat levels in the blood, which is good news for the heart.

98 BUTTER YOURSELF UP

It may be high in fat, but studies suggest that your body might be able to absorb more beneficial nutrients from vegetables when they are eaten with (a little) butter. They taste better, too!

98 SUBSTITUTE TEA FOR COFFEE

Tea, which is rich in polyphenols, has a protective effect on heart health, lowering blood pressure and helping heart health in the long term, particularly in older women.

miracle foods

100 BANANAS FOR MAXED-OUT NUTRIENTS

Bananas are rich in potassium, calcium, iron, magnesium and phosphorus. They are also a good source of vitamins A and C as well as the B vitamins thiamin, riboflavin and niacin. They contain all eight essential amino acids plus potassium, a potent brain fuel.

101 SPOON UP THE YOGURT

As well as helping balance beneficial gut bacteria, yogurt is rich in health-giving potassium, protein, riboflavin and vitamin B12. In addition, yogurt is a richer source of calcium than milk. Live yogurt cultures produce lactase, which break down lactose so it's good for lactose-intolerants.

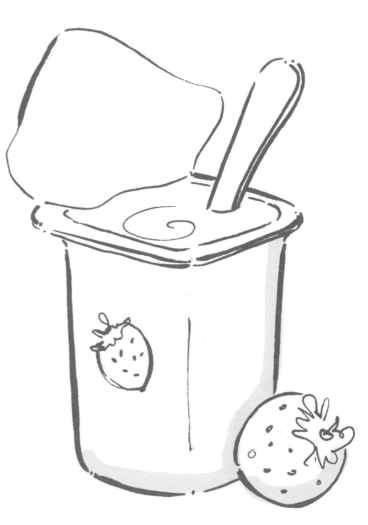

102 BROCCOLI FOR CALCIUM

This is a real miracle food. Just a single serving (1 cup raw) of broccoli contains 200% of the recommended daily amount (allowance) of vitamin C and 360mg of calcium. In addition, it has only 25 calories and just 0.3g of fat.

103 TRACK DOWN WILD SALMON

Wild salmon has as much as three times the amount of beneficial omega-3 oils as the farmed varieties, higher levels of the antioxidant astaxanthin and less fat, making it one of the best choices for healthy eating.

104 WHIP OUT THE WALNUTS

Walnuts are a superfood because they are rich in vegetable oils and beneficial fats,and they contain high levels of arginine, folate, fibre, tannins and polyphenols. They're an excellent way to boost protein intake, too.

105 GET YOUR OATS

Oats are one of the best sources of inositol, important for maintaining optimum blood cholesterol levels. They are also very high in soluble fibre and can help ease constipation. Unrolled oats release energy slowly into the body, making you stay fuller longer and so lessening any urge to snack.

106 YOU SAY TOMATO

Tomatoes are packed with lycopene, a disease-fighting antioxidant. One study found that 40mg of lycopene daily protects against heart disease, and smaller amounts may help, too. Cooked tomatoes and ketchup are the best sources.

107 EASE PAIN WITH CHERRIES

Cherries can relieve the pain of arthritis and gout. The ingredients that do the job, called anthocyanins, also act as antioxidants with an effect that is ten times more potent than vitamins E and C!

108 FIGHT DISEASE WITH BLUEBERRIES

Blueberries contain incredibly high levels of the antioxidant resveratrol – four times the amount found in cranberries or grapes. This makes the blueberry the ultimate food when it comes to fighting disease and boosting general health.

109 THE FUTURE IS ORANGE

Studies have shown that orange zest helps prevent the initiation and progression of breast cancer in rats and may also diminish the carcinogenic effects of tobacco. Add it to your daily diet to help prevent the risk of cancer – try fruit infusions or include zest in salad dressings.

110 STAY YOUNG WITH SOYA

Adding soya to your diet can help reduce the risk of ill health through heart disease, breast cancer and osteoporosis. Get your daily dose by substituting soya milk for cows' milk on breakfast cereals, in fruit smoothies or in your daily cappuccino.

111 TAKE TIME FOR TEA

Tea, although it contains caffeine, is highly beneficial for health. Green tea seems to break down fat in the body, while both black and green teas are rich in flavonoids, which destroy bacteria and viruses and protect against heart disease.

112 PICK PUMPKIN PIE

Pumpkin and pumpkin seeds are a very good source of potassium and sodium and contain a fair amount of vitamins B and C. Best of all, they are extremely high in vitamin A – 450g (1lb) of pumpkin can contain as much as 5,080 IU (international units), equivalent to 1.5mg RDA.

113 HAVE AN AVOCADO

Avocados are rich in vitamins A, B, C and E, as well as potassium. They have the highest protein content of any fruit and they are a rich source of monunsaturated fats, which are thought to lower blood cholesterol levels.

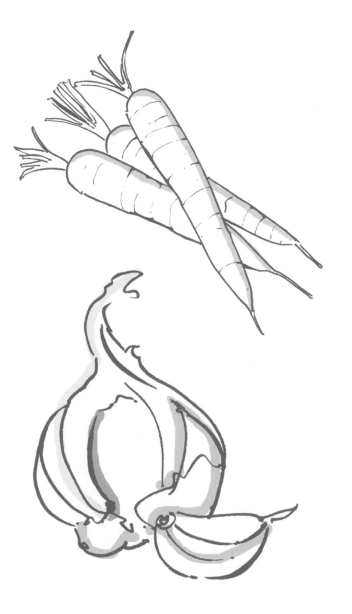

114 BUILD 24-CARROT BONES

If you want to build up the health of your bones without putting on any weight, then drink a glass of carrot juice every day. Carrot juice contains eight times as much calcium as milk, a host of other vitamins, and is packed with beneficial gut-regulating fibre.

115 PUT THE ONUS ON ONIONS

Onions, chives and spring onions (scallions) have a high sulphur content. Sulphur is a mineral that helps prevent skin problems such as ringworm, fungal infections, dry skin and rashes.

116 HELP YOURSELF TO HEARTY GARLIC

Although it might not be great for those intimate moments of passion, garlic is great for the health of your heart. It causes the body to release nitric oxide, which keeps arteries pliable and supple, boosting circulation and helping regulate blood pressure.

117 GRAB A GRAPEFRUIT FOR WEIGHT LOSS

Eating grapefruit really does help people lose weight, and could reduce the risk of developing diabetes. Researchers have found that people who include grapefruit in their diet lose weight faster, an effect they think may be due to high levels of digestive enzymes in the fruit.

118 EAT YOURSELF HAPPY

Choose foods that are high in the mood-boosting substance tryptophan, including bananas, turkey, milk, yogurt, tuna and chicken, to help you stay happy and content between meals.

119 BUY ORGANIC FOR HEALTHY ORGANS

Organically grown fruit and vegetables contain significantly higher levels of disease-preventing antioxidants than conventionally grown food. This means that they're not only better for your health, but they're also better for the overall environment.

120 MUNCH AWAY CANCER

Tomatoes, carrots and red peppers could help your body fight serious diseases like leukaemia by destroying cancerous cells. This is because they contain high levels of betacarotene, which has been shown in trials to encourage the death of cancerous cells in some forms of cancer.

121 APPLE EVER AFTER

Apples, grapefruits, cherries and apricots could be potent weapons in the war against cancer because of the high levels of d-glucarate they contain. The substance has been shown to decrease the risk of skin, liver, breast and colon cancers.

122 FISH FOR FITNESS

Already thought to prevent heart disease and other circulatory disorders by working against the degenerative processes of atherosclerosis, fish oils, which are rich in omega-3 fatty acids, may also play a role in boosting aerobic fitness.

123 CANCER-FIGHTING KUMQUATS

Eating citrus fruits, including the peel, helps in the fight against cancer. They contain chemicals called monoterpenes, including d-limonene, and have particular value in preventing breast, liver and lung cancers. Try kumquats, which you can eat rind and all.

salt

124 KNOW YOUR LIMITS

Scientists recommend that the average person keep sodium intake to no more than 2,400mg a day for healthy blood pressure. It might sound a lot, but this is only what you would get from a takeaway burger and a cup of chicken soup.

125 SEE CLEARLY NOW THE SALT IS GONE

Eating less salt can halve your risk of getting cataracts because high levels of sodium encourage development of the condition.

126 MAKE A HERBAL AGREEMENT

Instead of using salt, substitute herbs and spices, such as oregano, basil, coriander, thyme, parsley, cinnamon, nutmeg, cayenne pepper or paprika. Or season with lemon, garlic or vinegar.

127 BE SUSPICIOUS OF PREPARED SOUPS

Soup containing as much as 6.25g (¼oz) of salt per 250g (9oz) product has been found on sale on some supermarket shelves. This is about the same concentration of salt found in seawater. Look closely at sodium levels on processed and preserved foods before buying.

128 LOWER BLOOD PRESSURE WITH A LOW- SALT DIET

Low-salt diets have been shown to reduce blood pressure in people affected by elevated blood pressure. The diet alters the salt concentration of the blood, encouraging less water retention.

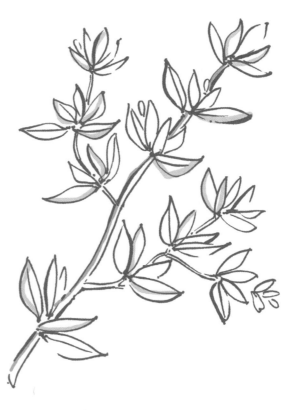

129 GARGLE TO TARGET ULCERS

Saltwater can help prevent infection by clearing up damaging bacteria, particularly in sensitive areas. Studies have shown that gargling or mouthwashing with saltwater can significantly speed up the healing of mouth ulcers.

130 DETOX WITH A SALTY SPA

Detox skin and help yourself relax by adding half a cup of sea salt to your bath as it fills up. Not only will it stimulate your skin, you'll float better in it, taking the strain off muscles.

131 SALTY SCRUB FOR BETTER CIRCULATION

Mix 2 cups of fine sea salt with 4 cups of grapeseed, apricot or almond oil and 20 drops of your favourite essential oil. Vigorously but gently massage into damp skin, beginning at the feet, in a circular motion. Avoid any scratched or wounded areas. The scrub will help your circulation and improve the texture of the skin.

sugars & fats

132 DON'T SWEETEN YOURSELF UP FOR OLD AGE

There is some evidence that consuming too much sugar can age your skin almost as much as smoking and sunbathing, by putting strain on the body's systems.

133 GO CANADIAN

Maple syrup is sweet and natural, with half the calories of normal sugar. For a healthy alternative to your usual sweetener, drizzle a few drops of maple syrup into tea or coffee or over desserts and discover its delicious and distinctive woody taste.

134 SHOW ME THE HONEY

Honey has fewer calories than sugar, it can help boost immunity and it is a good, natural alternative to refined sugars. If you're feeling under the weather, try manuka honey, made with pollen from the tea tree, famed for its healing powers.

135 BE A SUGAR DETECTIVE

Watch out for hidden sugars in low-fat foods such as soup, sauces and yogurts. Contents lists take sugars into account, so make sure you don't just look at the fat total on the label.

136 BEAT SUGAR FATIGUE

Fatigue could be due to fluctuations in blood sugar, which can cause metabolic changes in the body. Switch to slow-release sugars, such as fructose from fruit, to get your energy back.

137 EAT TO DRINK

Alcohol, especially if drunk with sugary mixer drinks, raises blood sugar and can lead to a blood sugar 'crash' later on, which is why people often feel hungry after a night out. The best foods to eat if you're hungry for a post-drink snack are ones that release energy slowly to regulate your blood sugar levels – oats, fruit, pasta and wholegrains.

138 DILUTE THE FRUIT

Fruit juices are high in sugar. If you're drinking them to start your day, why not try mixing them with about 5% water to aid absorption, prevent dehydration and rapid blood sugar fluctuations, and save calories as well?

139 AVOID THE POST-LUNCH SLUMP

If mid-afternoon tends to be your tired time, then it's possible you are overdosing on refined carbohydrates at lunch, which can cause your body to become carbohydrate sensitive. To overcome this, add more protein and fibre to meals and make sure you drink lots of water.

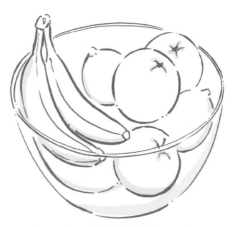

140 DON'T FALL FOR THE FAT TRAP

Calories in the form of sugar are just as fattening as calories in the form of fat – all excess calories are stored in the body as fat tissue, so don't fall into the low-fat, high-sugar trap.

141 CAN THE FIZZ

Just one can of carbonated soda can contain up to 35g (1¼oz) of sugar, as much as several packets of sweets. So the next time you feel like something bubbly, try sparkling mineral water instead.

vitamins

142 BAN THE ALUMINIUM PAN

If you're cooking vitamin-rich foods, stick to stainless steel, enamel or glass pans because pans made of aluminium and copper can react with sulphur compounds in vegetables to destroy vitamin C, folic acid and vitamin E.

143 KEEP OK WITH VITAMIN K

Vitamin K, found in leafy green vegetables, cheese, egg yolks, pork and liver, is essential to enhance bone formation and maintain bone density, especially in women.

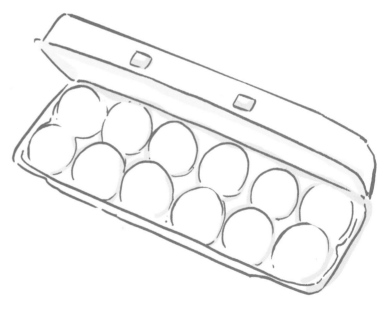

144 FOCUS ON FOLATE

Folate is not only essential for all-over body health, it's also a key ingredient for foetal development in the first three months of pregnancy. Get your dose from mushrooms, bananas, egg yolks, lentils, beans, peanuts, fortified breads and cereals, leafy green vegetables, romaine lettuce, oranges and other citrus fruits and juices.

145 SPRING CLEAN YOUR ARTERIES

Taking a supplement containing vitamins B12, B6 and folic acid could help prevent your arteries from getting blocked by lowering levels of artery-damaging homocysteine in the blood.

146 TAKE VITAMINS TO CATCH FREE RADICALS

Women need more antioxidants than men to mop up higher levels of free radicals and other negative elements in the female body. Vitamins C and E have been shown to maintain healthy arteries for heart health.

147 C OUT YOUR CENTURY

Vitamin C doesn't only reduce the risk of heart disease and other illness: it can also help you live longer. Studies have shown that people with high levels of vitamin C in their blood can increase the length of their life by several years.

148 COMBINE FOR BETTER HEALTH

Vitamins C and E exert a more powerful beneficial effect on women's health when taken in combination than separately, with the best health benefits seen in cognitive performance, memory and stroke prevention.

149 PROTECT AGAINST MS

High levels of vitamin D could help protect you against the development of multiple sclerosis (MS), especially if it is taken in quantities of more than 400 IU (international units) a day, which could slash risk by up to a third. Vitamin D is also known to help the body absorb calcium, essential for strong bones.

150 BE AN ACE THINKER

Vitamins A, C and E, as well as being powerful health-promoting antioxidants, can also help your mind stay sharp in old age by reducing your chances of suffering memory loss and Alzheimer's disease.

151 BREATHE EASY WITH E, A AND C

Vitamins A, C and E are essential for the best lung functioning, especially in young men and women, so to ensure you breathe easy for life, top up on these health-giving vitamins, found in fresh fruits and vegetables, fruit juice and supplements.

weight

152 THINKING THIN

The brain consumes about 20% of the body's energy intake, despite constituting only about 2% of its mass. So 15 hours of thinking could burn a whole gram of fat.

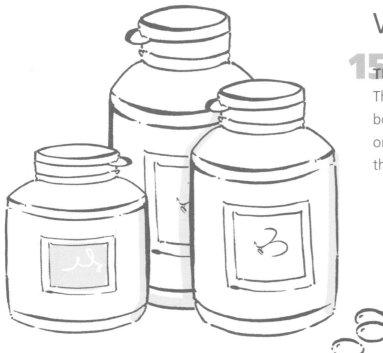

153 MEASURE YOUR WAIST WEIGHT

Measuring your waist will give you at least a rough guide to whether or not you need to lose some weight. For women taller than 1.52m (5ft), a waist measurement of more than 88cm (35in) is considered to be dangerous and they should seek help in losing weight.

154 DON'T GO TOTALLY TEE-TOTAL

When cutting calories, don't give up alcohol completely. Drink a glass or two of antioxidant-rich wine or beer a day because the anthocyanins and other antioxidants they contain can play a part in preventing 'bad' cholesterol from being deposited in blood vessels.

155 BIG-BOTTOM BENEFITS

Women who have pear-shaped bodies, carrying more weight on their hips and bottom, are at less risk of heart disease, diabetes and high blood pressure than their apple-shaped peers. Storing extra fat around the middle hinders the function of the organs. So be proud to be a pear.

156 DRINK UP TO FEEL FULL

Sipping water with food encourages the fibre in food to swell, making you feel fuller for longer. It also stimulates the liver to produce beneficial blood-cleaning fats, which moderate the rate and level at which your body absorbs fat and so help keep you looking slim.

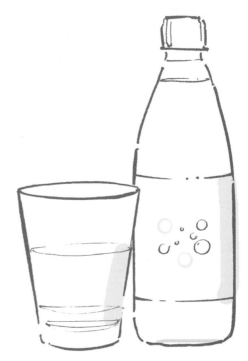

157 LOVE GARLIC TO LOSE WEIGHT

Garlic contains allicin, which prevents damaging cholesterol from being deposited in blood vessels and helps boost the removal of fats in the body.

158 EASE OFF ANIMAL FAT

Too many saturated animal fats can raise levels of bad cholesterol and lead to obesity. Keep intake sensible and try to consume them with fibre and water.

159 BE WARY OF WOLFING

Instead of wolfing down meals and snacks, take time to savour them. People who spend more time and attention on eating tend to eat less and avoid overeating.

160 PLAY CHOPSTICKS

Using chopsticks or swapping your knife and fork into the wrong hands will make you work harder to get the food into your mouth, which uses up more calories. It may also encourage you to take smaller bites.

161 THROW AWAY YOUR SCALES

One cell of muscle can weigh twice as much as a fat cell but takes up only half the amount of space. Relying less on the scales and more on how you actually look in the mirror or how your clothes fit could give you a far better picture of your all-round health.

162 SNIFF TO LOSE WEIGHT

Experts have shown that sniffing the scent of banana, green apples and peppermint can help people lose weight. Instead of snacking, try inhaling one or all of the scents to stave off hunger pains.

163 THINK OF THIRST FIRST

Feeling hungry? Make sure your body's not confusing thirst with hunger by drinking a glass of water before you start eating. Many of us have poor thirst mechanisms and may reach for food when we should be trying to get our optimum target of 2 litres (3½ pints) of water a day.

164 FIDGET AWAY FAT

Researchers believe extra movements burn up more calories. So in order to keep your body burning unwanted fat, always be on the move. Any extra body movements you can introduce into your normal day-to-day routine – from shifting your position more often than usual when sitting down, to occupying your hands when watching the television (whether you do this by playing with a stress-relieving toy or ironing the bed linen doesn't matter) will help you lose weight more easily. Try hiding the remote control (if you know where it is, of course) so you have to get up to change the channels or adjust the volume.

165 CHICORY LEAVES TO LOSE WEIGHT

Not only does chicory contain ingredients that could help you lose weight, it can also boost gut function by encouraging beneficial bacteria, helping prevent osteoporosis and protecting against gut and colon cancer.

166 DON'T BE A CORN BLOB

High-fructose corn syrup, of the type used as a sugar substitute in some processed foods, is thought to bypass the digestive processes and end up at the liver intact. This places extreme pressure on the health of the organ and it's thought that it could lead to diabetes.

167 EAT FAST, DIE YOUNG

Fast food could trick the body into eating more by containing up to three times as much energy per 100g (3½oz) than our bodies have evolved to cope with. By contrast, balanced meals fill us up without adding the extra calories.

168 KEEP DRINKING TO DROP WEIGHT

If you don't seem to be able to lose weight, or your diet has stopped showing results, check how much water you've been drinking. Water levels need to be kept high to keep the metabolism rate at weight-loss potential.

169 DO YOUR MATHS

Weight loss is a simple maths formula: 450g (1lb) of weight is equal to 3,500 calories, so you need to cut back by about 500 calories a day to lose 450g (1lb) a week.

170 WALK AWAY WEIGHT

Aim to do 30 minutes of moderate physical activity, where you feel slightly warm and out of breath, most days of the week. Brisk walking is ideal and will burn 150 calories.

171 DRESS LESS TO LOSE A SIZE

Salad might be the healthy option on many menus but just one teaspoon of salad dressing can hold 5g–10g of fat. Switch to oil-free or low-fat dressings to put your diet back on track.

172 CURB YOUR APPETITE WITH SOYA

Soya – especially if eaten raw – raises levels of the natural body hormone CCK, which reduces food intake by inducing a feeling of fullness and reducing appetite.

173 SLEEP YOURSELF SLIM

If you sleep for less than six hours a night, you could reduce your body's ability to burn off sugar, which means it is stored as fat instead. Make sure you sleep for seven to eight hours to stay slim.

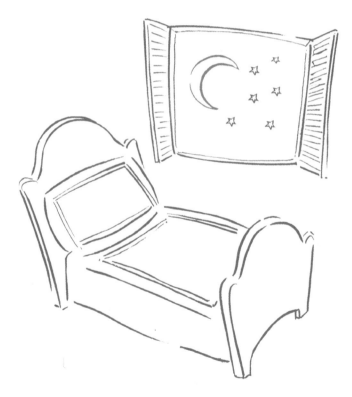

aromatherapy

174 SOAK AWAY YOUR BAD MOOD
Adding 3–5 drops of essential oil to a warm bath can either invigorate you or relax you, depending on the oil. Orange, grapefruit, ginger and peppermint are stimulating and will help you get going while lavender, geranium, rose and neroli are relaxing and calming.

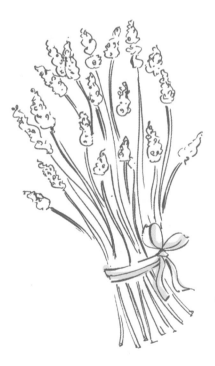

175 LIE DOWN WITH LAVENDER

Inhaling essential oil of lavender has been shown to have sedative and relaxing effects, so add a few drops to your pillow if you suffer from insomnia. It makes a perfect bedtime partner on hard-to-sleep nights.

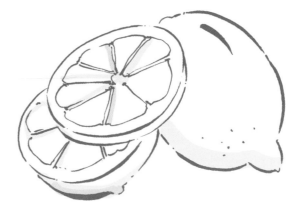

176 PLEASURE HIM WITH PUMPKINS

Experts have found that the odour produced by pumpkin can increase sexual arousal in men. Though it may sound like a strange aphrodisiac, if you're feeling frisky, get down to some home cooking and feed him a slice of pumpkin pie. Alternatively light a pumpkin-scented candle or use a pumpkin fragrance oil in potpourri.

177 GET SEXY WITH LIQUORICE LIPS

The scent of liquorice increases sexual stimulation in women, as does the scent of cucumber. Freshly chopped foods release the strongest scent, and the longest-lasting odour is usually found on or near the skin of fruit and vegetables rather than in the flesh.

178 ENHANCE EFFICIENCY WITH LEMON

The scent of lemons (and, to a lesser extent, other citrus fruits such as limes, grapefruits and oranges) could help boost efficiency in the workplace by making workers more alert and increasing their ability to concentrate.

179 PICK A PICK-ME-UP

The garden herbs basil and rosemary could mimic the effects of get-up-and-go hormones adrenaline and cortisol in the bloodstream, giving you extra energy to get through long days. Use them in cooking or use fresh or dried herbs to scent rooms.

180 CHILL OUT WITH ICE CREAM

Don't feel guilty about putting that extra spoon of vanilla ice cream in your bowl. Experts have shown that the smell of vanilla in drinks, food and atomizers helps people deal with stress.

181 SMELL TO SMARTNESS

Not only can aromatherapy help you become calm and relaxed, it could also boost the power of your brain. Researchers have found that the regular use of lavender and lemon balm oils slowed down the onset of dementia.

182 MASSAGE YOUR WAY TO HEAVEN-SCENT SKIN

An aromatherapy massage with German camomile and sandalwood can calm skin irritation and help endow your body and face with a healthy glow. For the best results, use a non-greasy carrier oil, such as almond or jojoba, and avoid delicate areas, especially the eyes.

balance

183 KEEP SKIN SILKY-SMOOTH

Exfoliating the skin to remove dead skin cells may help you retain a good sense of balance by heightening the sensation powers of your skin, thus allowing your body to make tiny adjustments.

184 GET FIT TO STAND TALL

Fitter people have better balance, not just because of their tendency to be the correct weight but also because their nerves and muscles are used to working together to keep their body upright.

185 BE A FLAMINGO FOR BETTER BALANCE

Practise standing on one leg, with your eyes fixed on a stationary spot in front of you. Start on a hard floor and progress to carpet or foam. Once you can stand balanced for a whole minute, try changing the positions of your arms, legs and eyes without falling over.

186 DON'T SPILL A DROP

Don't just drink eight full glasses of water a day – use them as an opportunity to work on your balance by walking around without spilling them for a few minutes before you take a sip.

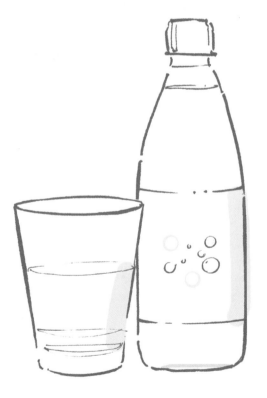

187 LOOK INSIDE TO CENTRE YOURSELF

Recent studies have revealed that those people who practise techniques that involve breathing exercises and inner contemplation – such as yoga, tai chi and chi gong – have better balance than those who don't.

188 AVOID CRACKS TO SPEED UP REACTIONS

Practise walking faster and stepping over or avoiding objects lying in your path, such as cracks in the pavement or tiles on the kitchen or bathroom floor. This will help improve the speed of your walking and decrease hesitancy.

189 GET BALANCED AS YOU GET OLDER

Balance problems affect more than a third of people over 65 years of age, and more than half of those aged over 75. Make certain that you prepare your balance muscles with regular exercises well before you reach this stage.

190 STAND UP SLOWLY TO HELP YOUR HEAD

Morning dizziness is often caused by a drop in blood pressure upon standing, particularly after a long time spent lying down. Get up slowly to give the blood time to work its way around the body.

193 GET A SENSE OF HUMMUS

Increasing fibre intake helps level out circulation by aiding fluid balance after eating. Pulse (legume) spreads like hummus and bean dips, in place of sour cream and cheese spreads or dips, are tasty ways to eat more fibre.

circulation

191 MAKE FRIENDS WITH FRUIT

People with high levels of fruit and vegetables in their diets have lower blood pressure than those who choose less healthy foods, probably thanks to good salt and sugar regulation.

192 GET UP TO SCRATCH WITH CAT'S CLAW

The herbal extract cat's claw, which comes from an Amazonian rainforest plant, has been shown to lower blood pressure in some clinical trials.

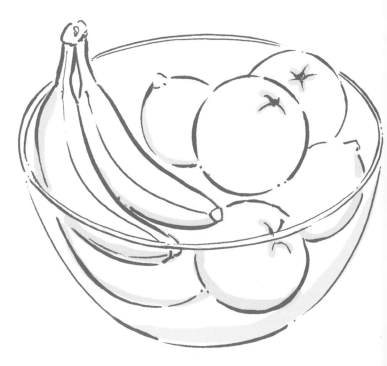

194 SPRINKLE AWAY STICKINESS

Vitamin E, which is found commonly in seeds like pumpkin and linseed (flax) and in fruits such as cherries, kiwi and green peppers, has been shown to reduce the stickiness of the blood, so reducing the possibility of clotting. Sprinkle the seeds on salads for a daily dose.

195 GO ORANGE FOR STRENGTH

Oranges and other types of citrus fruit contain high levels of vitamin C and bioflavonoids. These substances work in the body to strengthen the walls of capillaries to keep blood pumping fast around the body.

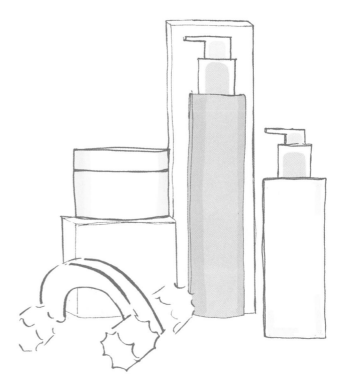

196 TAKE IT NIACIN EASY

Niacin, which is also known as vitamin B3 and is found in liver, poultry, pulses (legumes), nuts, cereals and rosehips, boosts the circulation and blood flow to the small blood vessels, helping alleviate circulation problems.

197 PRESS AWAY PROBLEMS

Massage has major benefits for circulation as it increases blood flow to the area being treated, increasing the flow of nutrient-rich, oxygenated blood to skin, muscles and underlying tissues.

199 SOCK IT TO 'EM

Wearing elasticated flight socks, particularly on air journeys of longer than about 90 minutes, can help blood return from the lower legs and so reduce the chances of DVT (deep-vein thrombosis) and dangerous blood clots developing.

200 HANG LOOSE TO STOP CLOTS

Body-hugging neoprene sports shorts, said to promote weight loss and designed for use in the gym or aerobics classes, may, however, increase the risk of blood clots developing in the legs by restricting blood flow. Choose looser clothes instead to safeguard your circulation.

201 GO FRUITY

Fruit that contains high levels of lycopene helps general circulation in the body by preventing a buildup of plaque, which restricts blood flow through arteries. A tasty choice is watermelon, which contains 14mg per slice.

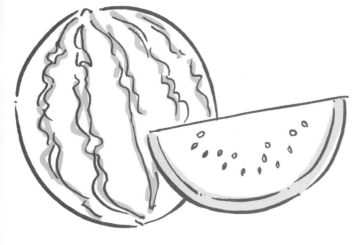

198 CURE COLD FEET WITH CAYENNE

Soaking feet and hands in water with a teaspoon of mustard powder or cayenne pepper for five to ten minutes can help boost circulation by dilating blood vessels.

202 WEED OUT THE WEED

Smoking is the single worst thing you can do for your circulation. It narrows arteries, breaks down capillary walls and stops the heart working efficiently. There's only one answer – give up.

203 GET TO THE POINT

Reflexology, a technique that concentrates on stimulating pressure points on the feet, can help boost blood flow to the feet and legs, hence improving circulation.

204 POUND AWAY PRESSURE

Working out at least three times a week boosts circulation, clears out arteries and lowers blood pressure, giving the circulation system an energy boost.

205 GET JIGGY WITH GINSENG

Extract of ginseng not only alleviates problems caused by bad circulation but increases blood flow to the extremities, boosting health and wellbeing.

206 STAND ON YOUR HEAD

Not for those with a health condition, head and shoulder stands boost circulation to the head and neck. For a safer alternative, try sitting with your head between your knees for several minutes.

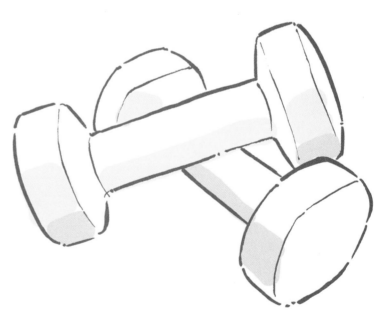

207 PUT YOUR FEET UP

Lounging about watching television for hours at a time or slumped in a chair reading can leave you in bad positions for blood drainage and impair lower-limb circulation as a result. By putting your feet up, however, you will place less stress on your system – and you might find that it's more comfortable, too!

208 POUND THE PAVEMENT

Any type of physical exercise that involve impact on the feet and hands – such as skipping, running, walking, boxing and kickboxing – improves circulation to the extremities. Impact exercise can also prevent pain and the onset of problems.

208 DETOX YOUR ARTERIES

Studies have shown that eating garlic can help reduce the buildup of plaque in arteries, and even clear away existing deposits. Aim to include some in your diet once a day or take a supplement.

core strength

210 COUGH UP A CORE

Your core strength relies on the muscles you use every time you cough. So, in order to find the muscles, cough gently a few times and use your fingers to feel where your abdomen contracts. These are the muscles that hold your trunk erect.

211 TILT INTO SHAPE

Try this pelvic tilt, which is proven to strengthen the abdominals. Lie on your back with knees bent and feet flat on the floor. Breathe out and draw your abdominals down towards your spine, hold, and repeat several times.

212 BRACE YOURSELF

Practise forming a 'back brace' by pulling your bellybutton inwards without flattening your back, then tightening your pelvic floor muscles as if you were stopping the flow of urine. Keep your breathing relaxed.

213 HAVE A BALL

Swiss ball exercises can help strengthen your spine and core muscles safely and easily. Try swapping the sofa for a ball as you watch television, or engaging your body fully by using one at your work desk instead of a chair.

214 SWING OUT SISTER

To boost core strength, stand beside a table or wall (in case you overbalance) and stand on one leg. Swing the outer leg backwards and forwards. Make sure you don't dip, twist or rotate your pelvis.

215 THINK YOURSELF STRONG

Hard to believe, but imagining yourself with strong core abdominal muscles could actually make them stronger by more than 10%. It's no substitute for exercise, but it's better than nothing!

216 BE STRAIGHT WITH YOURSELF

Try this simple exercise: stand up straight with your eyes closed and concentrate on feeling the muscles in your body adapting to keep you in position. This will help core strength as well as your balance.

217 WORK IT AT WORK

Don't allow yourself to fall into bad habits at work that can ruin your posture. For toning, and to remind yourself to stay strong at the core, contract your abdominals and pelvic floor muscles from time to time as you sit at your desk.

218 PULL IN YOUR BELLY TO PROTECT YOUR BACK

Having poor core strength makes you many times more susceptible to injury and lower-back pain, as the spine is forced into adopting unnatural positions. To support your lower back, pull your bellybutton upwards and backwards until you feel 'lifted'.

energy boosters

219 CRUNCH CRACKERS FOR GOOD SNACKING

Wholewheat or rice crackers spread with peanut butter, tahini, hummus or low-fat savoury spreads like tapenade have been shown to help weight loss and boost energy levels by curbing unhealthy snacking.

220 GO HOT FOR GET-UP-AND-GO

For an instant pick-me-up at mealtimes, dust your food with chilli powder, cumin and coriander. These spices are a natural and tasty way to invigorate your body, and there is no drawback of a corresponding sugar low afterwards.

221 HAVE A BRAZILIAN

No, not a bikini wax, but a healthy eating alternative instead! Brazil nuts not only boost short-term energy, but just three a day can also help cut the risk of heart disease by a third.

222 BE A SUNFLOWER SEEKER

Toasted sunflower seeds are a great choice to nibble on when afternoons at work begin to drag. Not only will they stop you reaching for fatty, salty snacks, they'll also boost your energy-giving vitamin levels while you munch.

223 APPRECIATE THE APRICOT

Dried apricots, perfect substitutes for biscuits (crackers) with cheese, are an excellent source of fibre, potassium, iron and betacarotene. Choose air-dried, not sulphur-dried, as sulphites have been linked to different forms of cancer.

224 STRETCH AND YAWN TO WORK OUT FACE MUSCLES

Stretching allows blood to flow into muscles that have become inactive, which is why it's so regenerating after sleep. Yawning gives your body a big oxygen boost, which combines with the stretching to give muscles instant energy.

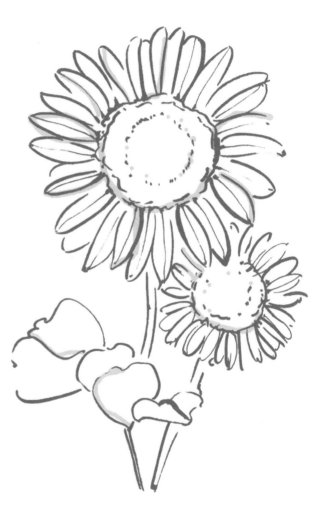

225 FEEL CHIPPER WITH BANANA

For a handy and tasty pick-me-up, why not try dried banana chips? They are rich in carbohydrates, iron and magnesium and, in addition, they have natural sugars to give your body an energy boost when you're on the move. Combine them with plain, natural yogurt when you're looking for a more substantial snack.

226 WAKE UP TO MORNING GLORY

For a morning boost, swap your first cup of tea or coffee for an energy-giving detox drink made with hot water, lemon juice, freshly grated ginger, maple syrup and a pinch of cayenne pepper.

227 LIQUIDIZE YOUR ASSETS

Make a natural power drink by liquidizing apples, banana and a tablespoon of peanut butter together. Drink a glass with your breakfast. The fruit sugars will boost your energy at different levels to keep you going all morning.

228 FEEL BLOOMING GOOD

Add a ray of natural sunshine to your life by feasting on edible flowers like violets, nasturtiums, marigolds, primroses and pansies, which can benefit body and mind.

eyesight

229 LOOSEN UP FOR AN EASY VIEW

Tight collars and ties have been shown to raise blood pressure in the eyes, which is a leading risk factor in glaucoma, by constricting the jugular vein. If your neck's under pressure, loosen up!

230 FISH OILS FOR NIGHT VISION

Problems with night vision can be relieved by adding extra essential fatty acids (EFAs) from fish oils to your diet. Deficiencies can also lead to retinal damage. So if you want to see in the dark, make sure you eat at least two portions of oily fish a week.

231 STOP DEGENERATION WITH VITAMIN A

Very high doses of vitamin A may provide a cure for age-related macular degeneration, which is a very common cause of blindness in the over-50s. The minimum effective dosage is currently being researched, since too much vitamin A can damage the liver. Consult your doctor for advice.

232 DON'T SALT UP YOUR SIGHT

Too much salt in your diet could double your risk of developing cataracts. Studies have shown that people who eat the least salt are the least likely to develop the condition. Watch out for hidden salts in processed foods, soups and cereals.

233 KEEP AGEING EYES IN THE CAN

Eating canned tuna more than once a week reduces the risk of developing age-related macular degeneration by more than 40%. Combine with vitamin-rich sweet potato and tomato for the best benefits.

234 TREAT YOURSELF TO A BERRY GOOD VIEW

Compounds called flavonoids, found in berries, protect the sensitive cells of the eye, which are especially prone to strain from work at computers. Drink a blueberry smoothie for a bright-eyed day.

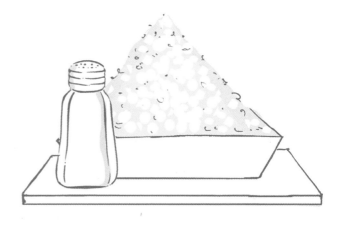

235 LOOK YOURSELF IN THE EYES

If the whites of your eyes appear dull or yellowish in colour, this could be an indication of a struggling liver. Help it out with milk thistle, ginger and citrus fruits.

236 COOK UP A GREAT VIEW

Carrots really can help you see in the dark. This is because the high levels of vitamins (especially vitamin A) they contain help protect eyes from daily wear and tear. The beneficial effects of carrots are easier to assimilate in the body if they're cooked (but not overcooked).

237 FOCUS ON FISH

Omega-3 fish oils are thought to protect the macula lutea (the spot at the centre of the retina) from problems. Aim to eat oily fish like tuna, mackerel or salmon more than once a week and use linseed (flaxseed) and sunflower oils for cooking.

238 KEEP ON THE LEVEL

Staring at a computer screen all day can be very damaging for the eyes, especially if the screen is badly positioned. Screens should be roughly 60cm (2ft) away with the top at eye level, and arms should rest lightly on the desk's surface.

239 EAT SWEET POTATO FOR SWEET VISION

Although they taste rich and creamy, sweet potatoes are fat- and cholesterol-free and full of vision-boosting betacarotene and vitamin A. One medium-sized sweet potato has only around 130 calories.

240 RETAIN AN EGG-CELLENT RETINA

Taurine, found in eggs, meat and fish, is an essential ingredient for keeping the retina strong and supple, enhancing vision.

241 CHOCOLATE FOR FIRST-RATE VISION

A daily dose of chocolate, particularly the dark, high cocoa-solids varieties, can help vision by topping up copper levels.

242 CUT OUT WHEAT AND BANISH UNDEREYE CIRCLES

Dark circles under the eyes, usually considered a sign of tiredness, can also be caused by food intolerance, often to refined foods. Try cutting out processed foods for a few days and see if they lighten up.

243 PUT YOUR EYES IN THE SHADE

The optician's no. 1 tip for healthy eyes is to make sure your sunglasses have high UVA and UVB protection, which will protect eyes against the damaging rays generated by the sun. This is guaranteed to give you a brighter future.

244 GIVE YOUR EYES A REST

Even if you have only a minute to spare, focus on something far away, blink several times to build up moisture, then hold the lids closed for a few seconds, pressing your palms over the sockets to rest and rejuvenate the eyes.

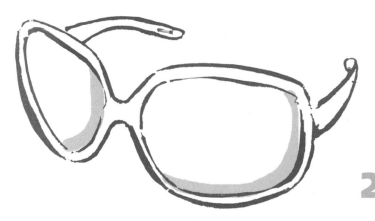

fertility

245 SAY NO TO SOYA

Food products that contain soya or that are wrapped in plastics may reduce the sperm count in men, as they may have chemicals that mimic the action of female hormones.

246 AXE THE ALCOHOL

Studies show that women who drink small amounts of alcohol (fewer than five units a week) double their chance of conceiving within six months compared with women who drink more.

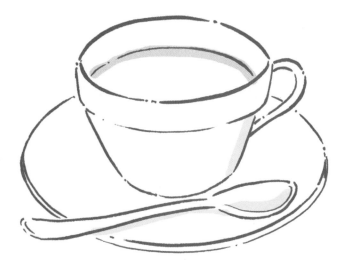

247 COUNT TEN TO CONCEPTION

Women wishing to conceive should make love every other day for a ten-day period during the middle of their cycle. Studies have shown that the five days before and the five days after the projected ovulation date are the most promising times to become pregnant.

248 RAISE A CUP TO FERTILI-TEA

Taking an infusion from 125g (4oz) or more of tea each day could double, or even in some cases triple, your chances of conception. Black teas contain slightly more caffeine than green, but either will do the trick.

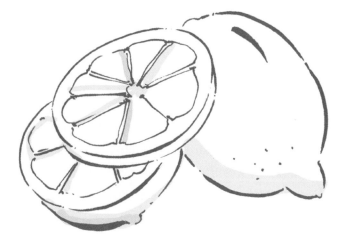

249 DON'T BE A LEMON

Calming coffee-free drinks like hot water with lemon juice may actually harm chances of conception because lemon juice has been shown to kill sperm, not only directly but also by altering the acid levels in the body.

250 WAIT UNTIL THE YEAR'S OUT

It is not unusual for most women to have to wait several months before conceiving, especially if they have been on the contraceptive pill for a number of years. Experts suggest that there is no need to worry about fertility until you've been trying for a year with no results.

251 DESTRESS TO BOOST EGG QUALITY

You can improve the quality of your eggs by cutting down on the stress in your life, which causes the body to release stress hormones such as adrenaline. These substances alter the natural hormone balance in the body and jeopardize the quality of eggs.

252 CONCEIVE WITHOUT COFFEE

High-caffeine products with none of tea's antioxidant benefits, like filter coffee, cola and energy drinks, have been shown to reduce the chances of conception in both men and women.

253 GIVE A FIG

Dried figs and apricots, wheatgerm, leafy green vegetables, sesame seeds and nuts are all good sources of magnesium, low levels of which have been shown to reduce the chances of conception in women.

254 ACCURATE PREGNANCY TESTING

Don't test too soon. One week after your expected period is the best time to take a pregnancy test. About 25% of women who ultimately get positive results, won't tests positive on the first day they miss their period.

immunity boosts

255 GRAB A GRAPE

Grapes, especially those with seeds, could boost immunity by inducing the production of important cells known as T-cells, which play a key part in protecting against viruses and bacteria in the body.

256 NATURE'S WAY

Natural immunity is something we're born with, but it can be boosted early in life by being breast-fed. Breast-feeding enables antibodies to be passed from the mother to the child.

257 SHORT-TERM BOOSTS

Echinacea – available as tablets or a liquid – stimulates phagocytosis, the consumption of invading organisms by white blood cells. The herb has maximum effect when taken in short courses to fight recurring infections, such as colds. For this reason, avoid taking it as a long-term preventive measure.

258 CHINESE HERBS FOR HEALTH

The Chinese herb astragalus stimulates immune-system activity by increasing the number of stem cells in the marrow and lymph, and stimulates their development into active immune cells. Research suggests that it can also trigger immune cells from a 'resting' phase into an 'active' phase.

posture

259 IF AT FIRST YOU DON'T SUCCEED...

Practise really does make perfect. It might sound staggering, but you may have to repeat a postural change around 10,000 times before it becomes sufficiently engraved on your brain to become a subconscious action.

260 DON'T LET SHOULDERS CREEP UP ON YOU

A common fault is to let shoulders creep up towards your ears as muscles tighten and the back bends forward. Gently hold shoulders back and try to keep space around the sides of your neck.

261 SUMMON SOME LUMBAR SUPPORT

Lumbar support should fit snugly into your spine at the point where it curves inwards at the waistband. If it is too low, it can put pressure on the sacroiliac joints, pushing the pelvis forwards.

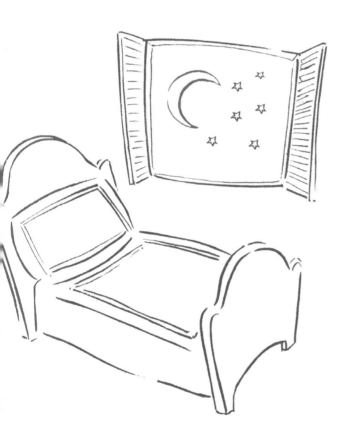

262 WALK TALL TO FREE YOUR BACK

As you walk around, lift your head until you're looking straight ahead of you, with a relaxed neck and shoulders. Press your shoulders back (not up) so your chest is pushed out, and straighten your spine so you are standing straight, but not too rigidly, like a ramrod.

263 KEEP CIRCULATION HEALTHY WITH THE THREE-FINGER GAP

If your feet are hanging or tucked under when you sit down, the increased pressure on the backs of the legs can impair return circulation from the feet. This can lead to or aggravate swollen ankles and varicose veins. Keep both feet on the floor and aim for no more than a a three-finger gap behind your knees.

264 GET FIRM AT NIGHT

Make sure your mattress is firm enough to support the contours of your body, to reduce pressure on the spine.

265 PULL YOUR KEYBOARD CLOSER

By holding your elbows away from your body you set up continuous tension in the muscles of the neck and shoulders, thus creating a buildup of lactic acid and other unwelcome by-products. If you're typing, make sure the keyboard is positioned so that your elbows fall to your sides, not in front of you.

266 SLEEPING SUPPORT

If you lie on your side in bed at night, consider putting a pillow between your knees to keep them at the same width as your hips, and so reduce twisting and strain on the pelvis. This will also help you avoid the discomfort of hip pain.

267 GIVE IT THE ELBOW

By bending your arms at the elbow when you walk, and using them to work your stride pattern, you will burn at least 5%–10% more calories than if you let them hang by your side.

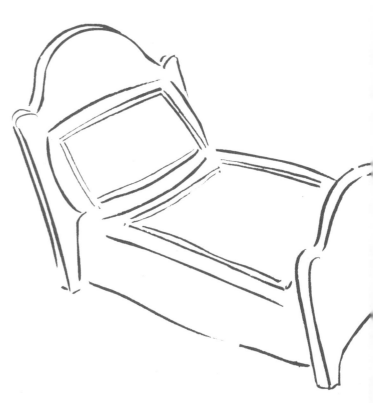

268 DON'T STRETCH TO FIT

For perfect posture, your neck should not be straight or stretched, but it should retain its slight natural curve with your chin parallel to the floor, neither tucked in nor jutting out.

269 IMAGINE A GOLDEN STRING TO BETTER POSTURE

This health tip is borrowed from the Alexander Technique, and it is a way to help you walk taller without injury. Imagine there is a golden string running vertically up your body through your spine, stretching you upwards through the crown of your head and creating space between each vertebra.

270 MAKE SLEEP A SIDE ISSUE

People who sleep on their side take an enormous amount of pressure off their spine compared with those who lie on their front or back. Lying face down is the worst position for overnight spine health.

271 LOOK AHEAD TO LOOK SHARP

It might be tempting to look at your feet as you walk along, but for the best posture you should focus on an imaginary spot about 3.5m–6m (12ft–20ft) in front of you. If your head is down, this increases strain on the neck and shoulders.

272 WALK FASTER, NOT LONGER

It is counterproductive – and potentially harmful to your back – to increase the length of your stride unnaturally. Speed and efficiency in walking are generated by hip flexibility and using quicker, not longer, steps.

273 STRETCH YOUR NECK TO RELEASE STRESS

Stand up straight with your back against a wall. Keeping your head level, without looking up or down, jut your neck forward. Then bring your chin straight back as if on railway tracks. Repeat five times to release tense neck muscles.

pressure points

274 GIVE YOURSELF A HELPING HAND

Your LI4 pressure point is located on the top side of the hand, between your thumb and your index finger. To locate it, squeeze the thumb against the base of the index finger. The point you are looking for is located on the highest point of the bulge of the muscle. Press this point for about 30 seconds to induce calmness and for a health-inducing digestive detox. However, you should not try this technique if you are pregnant.

275 PUT YOUR BEST FOOT FORWARD

Your L3 pressure point is found on the foot, on the line running between the big toe and the second toe and about three finger widths from the edge in the hollow on the top of the foot. Move your index finger anticlockwise over this point in order to induce relaxation and to unblock any anger and depression.

276 COMPRESS THE WRIST TO REDUCE THE STRESS

Find the spot between the tendons of the inside of the wrist, three finger widths from the palm. Breathe in, press as you breathe out slowly and repeat several times to reduce stress and strain.

277 CLEAR YOUR KIDNEYS

Your kidney point, which can be used to treat fatigue and lethargy as well as to detox the body through the kidneys, is located on the sole of the foot, just to the side of the ball of the foot under the second or third toe. Press and release several times.

278 ENJOY AN EXTRA ENERGY BOOST

Stimulating your stomach point can give you extra energy when you're flagging or tired. It is located just below the knee, on the outside of the shinbone. Press for at least 30 seconds with the pad of your finger or thumb.

278 TEND TO NECK TENSION

A tension-relief point, good for reducing pain caused by tension headaches and relieving tired eyes, is found in the occipital hollow, where the bottom of the skull meets the neck on either side of the spine. Use a thumb on either side to compress this area but be very careful not to press too hard.

280 ARM YOURSELF AGAINST ANXIETY

A stress-relieving point for reducing anxiety and tension is found at the top centre of the forearm (with palm facing down) in the large section of muscle just underneath the crease of the elbow. Press for several seconds and release several times.

281 LISTEN TO YOUR HEART

Your SI19 point is located near the ear, just before the small projection in front of the ear canal. It's in the depression that forms when the mouth is opened. Press for several seconds to release your inner emotions and desires.

282 STEP UP TO BOOST METABOLISM

A metabolism-boosting point is found on top of the foot, roughly in line with the middle two toes and directly over the arch. Use two fingers to apply broader pressure here because of the bones and ligaments.

283 GET IMMEDIATE IMMUNITY

An immunity-boosting point that is also good for combating fatigue, depression and general feelings of sluggishness is found on the inside of the ankle above the foot between the Achilles tendon and the ankle bone. Press and release several times for 10–20 seconds.

284 FORM A FIST TO HELP A HEADACHE

A point for general pain relief (especially of headaches) is found on the back, in line with the kidneys. The best way to stimulate this point is to sit up straight on a chair and form a fist with both hands. Place the fists behind your back so they touch and lie level with the elbow. Lean back gently.

285 DO AN ANTISTRESS PRESS

Stimulating the acupressure point that is located in the soft V-shaped area of flesh found between the thumb and forefinger can help reduce stress. Press the pad of your thumb into this area for at least 30 seconds and then repeat the same action on the other hand.

self-massage

286 GET IT OFF YOUR CHEST

In order to reduce tension across the front of the chest area, and to free up your breathing and loosen stress in your neck, place the four fingers of your right hand on the left side of your chest, underneath the clavicle bone. Move the fingers in circular motions, working outward towards the shoulder joint in deeper strokes. Repeat on the other side. Breathe in and out slowly as you massage.

287 HEAD OFF TENSION

To reduce tension in the scalp, spread out the fingers and thumbs of both hands and place them on either side of your head with the thumbs towards the back of the neck. Work in small circular motions, and then, after a few seconds, move the hands so they cover a different area.

288 STICK YOUR NECK OUT

To reduce neck tension, move the four fingers of your right hand in circular motions over the top of your left shoulder, turning your head to the right to stretch the muscles and ligaments at the front of the neck. Repeat on the other side.

289 DRAW TENSION FROM YOUR JAW

To relieve tension in your jaw and the sides of your face, place the four fingers of your left hand together on the jaw so the index finger fits into the bony area in front of the earlobe. Using small circular motions, work lightly, being careful not to press too hard.

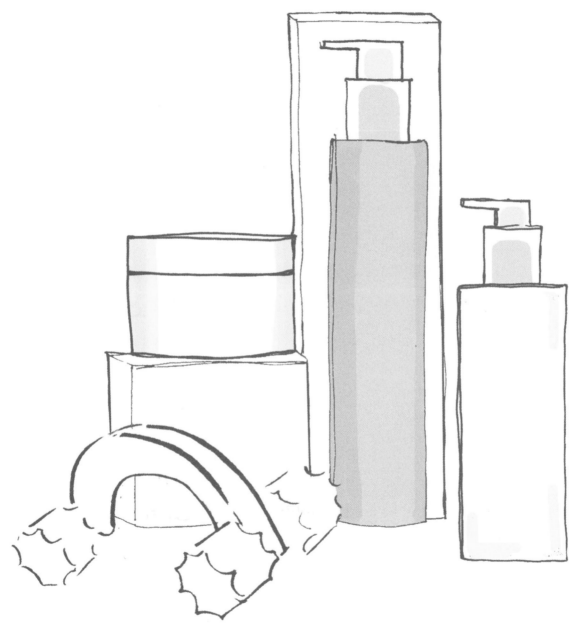

sense & sensation

290 LISTEN TO YOUR TASTEBUDS

If grapefruit is too bitter for you, you could be a supertaster. Supertasters average 425 tastebuds per square centimetre on the tips of their tongues, compared with 184 for most people.

291 EAT BEFORE YOU GET TOO HUNGRY

Hungry people taste salt and sugar more strongly than people who aren't hungry, so to avoid those salt and sugar cravings don't go for long periods without eating – have a healthy snack before you feel ravenous.

292 DON'T IGNORE YOUR FEMALE INTUITION

It's far from being a myth. Studies have shown that women who listen to their sixth sense are happier and healthier than those who ignore underlying feelings.

293 ADOPT A SENSE OF THE DAY

To make the most of your senses, pick a sense every day and make the most of it by fine-tuning. Concentrate on the everyday sensations you usually ignore to become more attuned to good sensations.

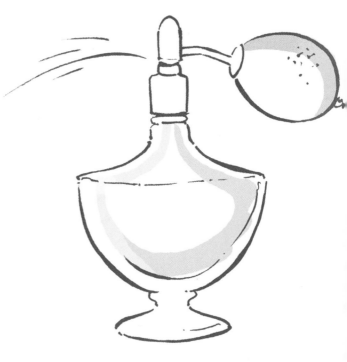

294 BECOME A CHILD EXPLORER

Children explore their environments with all of their senses – taste, smell, touch, sight and sound. So the next time you go somewhere new, don't rely just on sight and sound but think about how your other senses react as well.

295 DON'T NEGLECT YOUR MOST IMPORTANT SENSE

One of our senses is far and away the most important of all for health and happiness – so whatever you do and wherever you are, don't forget your sense of humour. People who can see the funny side of difficulties and problems are quicker at bouncing back from adversity.

296 LOOK AT YOUR FOOD

Without smell, our sense of taste would be next to nothing, but many people don't know that the look of food is important for taste as well. Food that looks good, quite simply, tastes good too.

sleep

297 SLEEP TO SURVIVE

Sleep could be as important as food for survival. Scientists have shown that animals deprived of sleep die within two to three weeks, almost the same length of time as if deprived of food.

298 JUICE UP TO DRIFT OFF

Juice together 3 apples, 2 oranges, 1 lemon and 2 handfuls of iceberg lettuce leaves (which contains lactones, calming substances that act as a natural sedative). Drink a glass before bed to help you sleep like a baby.

299 WATCH OUT FOR THE BURNOUT

If you feel tired during the day but can't sleep at night, it could be a sign that you're overtraining and not giving your body the rest it needs to thrive. If you don't feel motivated and alert within ten minutes of starting your workout, stop.

300 TRYP OFF TO SLEEP

Tryptophan is one of the eight essential amino acids obtained in the diet from protein foods such as milk and meat. It enhances sleepiness and stimulates the production of sleep-inducing hormones in the brain.

301 HOLD YOUR TONGUE

Experts suggest that you try this clever sleep trick to help you drop off: close your eyes and hold your tongue so it's not touching your cheeks or the roof of your mouth, as if you're yawning with your mouth closed. You'll be sleeping like a log in no time.

302 BE A HERBAL HIBERNATOR

Certain herbs such as valerian, camomile, hops and lime tree flowers have been shown to have sedative properties and are often taken either internally as a herbal tea or used within herbal pillows to enhance sleep.

303 SNACK ON SWEETCORN FOR A SLEEPY NIGHT

Some foods – including sweetcorn, oats, rice, tomatoes and bananas – contain traces of melatonin, which helps regulate sleep.

304 BEAT SNORING BY SLEEPING MORE

Sleep deprivation, especially if it's over several weeks, causes the muscles of the throat to sag, which leads to more snoring and less sleep. To stop snoring, aim for at least seven hours of sleep a night.

305 SLEEP TO STAY FIT

Cardiovascular function can be reduced by an astounding 11% after cumulative sleep deprivation, which means sleep is essential if you want to stay fit and healthy.

306 GO WITH THE FLOW

There's some evidence that reduced blood flow to hands and feet can keep you awake. Keep feet warm by wearing socks in bed or by investing in a hotwater bottle.

307 PUT SLEEP FIRST

Lack of sleep impairs your coordination, judgement and immune system, say the experts, so put sleep first for a healthy life and get into good habits by going to bed at about the same time every night. If a particular job or task isn't done by bedtime, just leave it until tomorrow.

308 BE A SLEEPING BEAUTY

Overnight, while you are asleep, your skin, hair and nails get a chance to regenerate themselves and deal with any health problems. Reducing the amount of sleep you get will therefore reduce the health of everything about your body, including the way you look.

309 BEWARE OF KNOCKOUT MEDICATIONS

Some medications used to treat insomnia may increase sleep, but if they reduce healing REM sleep you won't get the benefit of sleeping longer. Consult your doctor for advice.

310 SOAK AWAY INSOMNIA

A warm bath before bedtime can help you sleep by relaxing muscles and encouraging inactivity, which is essential for sleep. Try using calming aromatherapy oils such as lavender and lowering the lighting for an even sleepier experience.

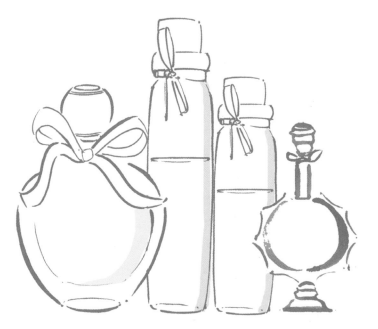

311 DON'T EXERCISE LAST THING AT NIGHT

Because undertaking physical exercise raises internal body temperature, which, in turn, wakes you up, exercising before bedtime is not a good way to tackle insomnia. Instead, try relaxing stretches or an indulgent bath.

312 KEEP YOUR SLEEP ON SCHEDULE

According to the experts, going to sleep at about the same time every night helps your body get into a regular sleep rhythm, which will help put a stop to any sleep problems. Similarly, try to get up at the same time every day in order to keep your schedule on track.

313 AVOID CAFFEINE AFTER DARK

Caffeine has well-known stimulant effects and drinking it before bed is likely to impair the quality of your sleep. Remember that chocolate contains caffeine, too, so that late-night treat might not in reality be a good idea either.

314 DON'T SPEED INTO SLEEP

If you are one of those people who fall asleep the very second their head hits the pillow at night, you could be suffering from the first effects of sleep deprivation. Healthy sleepers take an average of ten minutes to drop off.

315 SLEEP TO REGENER-EIGHT

It is estimated that the average person needs eight hours' sleep a night to re-energize body and mind, so don't beat yourself up about that weekend lie-in – your body needs it!

316 AIR YOUR SHEETS TO REFRESH YOUR SLEEP

Bacteria, mites and bedbugs thrive in moist conditions, so after you get up in the morning and instead of making the bed immediately, turn back the covers to allow the sheets to breathe for 30 minutes. Airing your bedroom by opening a window will help, too.

317 SLEEP LONGER TO LIVE LONGER

Recent studies have shown that people who sleep for less than six hours a night have a much higher mortality rate than those who give themselves just an hour or so longer in bed. So if you want to live longer, stay in bed.

318 SAY HIGH CARB FOR HIGH SLEEP

Glucose provides fuel for your brain, which is just as important while you are sleep as when you are awake. Eating foods that are rich in carbohydrates in the evening, especially those that release their sugar content slowly, helps promote long and healthy sleep.

319 SINK INTO EGYPTIAN COTTON

Egyptian cotton sheets wick away about 18% more moisture than other types of bedding. This not only leaves your skin healthy and dry, it also prevents moisture problems developing and increases overnight comfort.

320 BANISH INSOMNIA WITH ELVIS'S CURE

Elvis's favourite treat, the peanut butter and banana sandwich, could also be the best bedtime snack because of the high levels of sleep-inducing tryptophan it contains. It also releases energy slowly, promotIng healthy sleep cycles.

321 DON'T NAP AWAY YOUR NIGHT'S SLEEP

Napping can ruin sleep habits, so keep it down to 20 minutes and don't leave it until late – mid-afternoon is the best time.

322 HAND CARE WHILE YOU SLEEP

Not only does lavender hand cream give hands and nails a well-deserved moisture boost but its scent induces deep sleep.

323 SLEEP ON YOUR PROBLEMS

If you're living a stressful life, sleep might be the only chance your brain gets to sort out problems. The unconscious workings of your brain could mean you wake up in the morning with a surprise solution.

324 BE A COOL SLEEPER

Body temperature should drop naturally at night for the soundest, deepest sleep. Keep your bedroom cooler than the rest of the house and don't use covers you don't need. Research indicates that 16°C (62°F) is most conducive to restful sleep while temperatures above 24°C (71°F) are likely to cause restlessness.

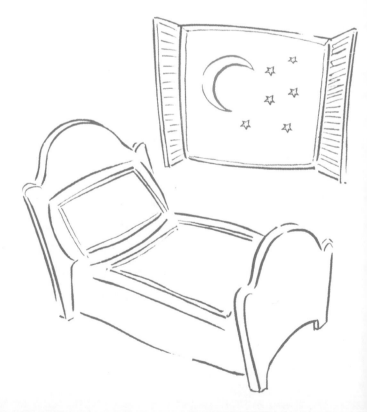

325 SLEEP TO STAY SLENDER

A lack of sleep could slow down your metabolism, causing your body to hold onto weight. To stay slim and keep your metabolism optimal, make sure you are getting at least seven hours of good-quality sleep every night.

workout wisdom

326 DRINK UP TO WORK OUT

Because water is essential to maximize metabolism, you won't reap the full benefits from your exercise routine unless you stay hydrated throughout. You can boost your body's performance on workouts simply by keeping topped up with water. Studies have shown that just a 3% loss in body fluid can lead to a 7% reduction in overall physical performance, so drink plenty of water before, during and after your workouts.

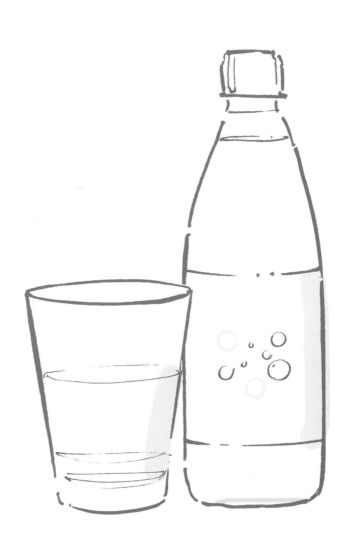

327 STRETCH IT OUT

Studies have suggested that stretching before undertaking exercise isn't as important as stretching afterwards. Instead, warm up at a slow pace beforehand and devote more time to stretching properly when you have finished.

328 GET INTENSE

High-intensity workouts have a greater and longer-lasting effect on increasing your resting metabolic rate, essential for long-term fat burning. Researchers have found that upping the intensity when you work out could help you burn as much as 300 extra calories a day, even at rest.

329 DO EXERCISE TO AVOID DIABETES

Exercise reduces fat tissue in the body and makes cells more responsive to insulin. Exercising five times a week has been shown to reduce the risk of diabetes by 45%, two to four times a week by 40% and once a week by 25%.

330 EAT MEAT TO BUILD MUSCLE

Meat-eaters who exercise regularly are more likely to build muscle, lose fat and tone up than their vegetarian counterparts, probably as a result of the higher levels of protein in the diet.

331 DON'T STARVE IF YOU WANT TO STAY FIT

People who don't feed their body enough fuel in the form of carbohydrates and proteins can't reach the same exercise intensities as others and therefore don't achieve the same metabolic changes or weight loss with exercise.

332 USE FRUIT FORCE

Snacking on healthy fresh or dried fruits, which contain slow-release fructose, teamed with a glass of milk after your exercise routine could improve long-term fitness and performance by rebuilding carbohydrate levels in the body, helping to metabolize fat.

333 BELT UP TO CURE SIDE PAIN

If you often suffer side stitches when you exercise, wearing an exercise belt could prevent pain. Raising your arms above your head or pressing the affected area for several minutes could also help.

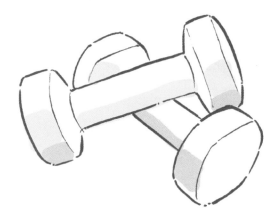

334 BREATHE IN, BREATHE OUT

Keep breath flow steady to nourish your body with oxygen. As a rule, inhale on the easy part of an exercise and exhale on the hard part to keep optimum oxygen levels.

335 STEP IT UP IN STYLE

Don't crank up the resistance on the Stairmaster or step machine so high that you have to lean on the arm posts, because this reduces efficiency. Instead, pump with your legs, get your heart rate up and progress slowly as you feel more comfortable with each level.

336 BE A VARIETY PERFORMER

For most of us, doing the same workout routine daily can induce boredom, not only in your head but also in your body, as it adapts to tasks. So vary your workouts and type of exercise to boost mental and physical fitness.

337 SCORE A GOAL OF THE MONTH

Set small, realistic goals – don't set yourself up for failure by aiming for unachievable targets. Decide on small goals you can achieve, such as three 30-minute sessions at the gym each week, which make it easier to experience success.

337 CATCH A WAVE TO TONE YOUR THIGHS

If you're not into sweating it out in gyms or taking up a team sport, but want to tone your legs the best way possible, get yourself a surfboard and catch a wave. Surfing is great for toning legs and abdominals as well as honing balance.

338 GIVE YOURSELF A GOLD MEDAL

Reward yourself for your successes. When you don't feel like exercising, remember how good you felt after exercising the last time, and reward yourself with healthy treats such as exercise clothes, new music to work out to or a sports massage.

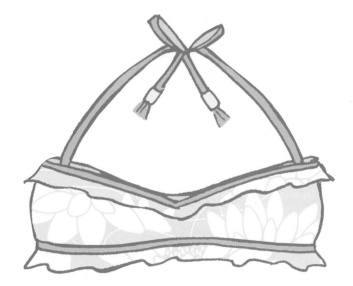

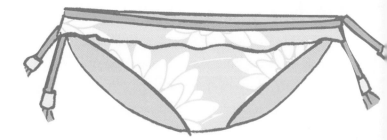

340 PUT YOUR BACK INTO IT

When devising a complete exercise plan, don't forget back exercises – although they might not seem as important as those showy triceps curls or leg squats, a strong back is absolutely key to effective, injury-free training.

341 POSTURE-PERFECT WORKOUTS

As you work out, don't forget to engage your core strength muscles in your abdomen, which will keep your trunk strong and steady and help you avoid succumbing to injury, as well as preventing bad exercise habits.

342 DON'T CURL UP TO SIT UP

Many people don't really work their abdominals properly during their situp exercise routines. Make sure you are moving the top of your body towards the ceiling, rather than curling it up towards your knees, which doesn't work the muscles as hard.

343 ANYONE FOR TENNIS?

Tennis burns 400 calories an hour and although it might not be such a good cardiovascular exercise as running or swimming, the tactical thinking stimulates your mind as well as your body, giving you a true holistic workout.

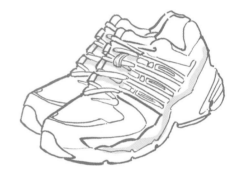

344 SQUASH UP YOUR BACKSIDE

Played competitively, squash will really firm up your arms and abdominals, as well as giving your system a cardiovascular boost. But it is also one of the best exercises around for toning up those flabby behinds because of all the lunging around court that is involved.

345 EXPLODE FOR STRENGTH

Explosive exercises – such as lunging – boost strength much faster than other types of weight training. To test this out, try doing your normal exercises more slowly, but with a high-impact beginning and ending.

346 SADDLE UP TO RIDE AWAY SADDLE BAGS

Horse-riding not only tones hips, legs and thighs through a series of leg exercises as you ride, it also increases strength and flexibility in your pelvis, hips and lower back, and works the thigh muscles to reduce fat.

347 ADD A FOOT OF TEXTURE

Simply wearing textured insoles inside sports shoes could help prevent knee and ankle injuries by increasing people's awareness of the position of their feet, particularly in fast-response sports like soccer and basketball.

348 SLAM DUNK THAT STOMACH FLAB

Basketball might be better known for toning arms and legs than stomachs, but all that twisting and stretching for the basket is, in fact, one of the best ways to get rid of stomach flab, especially if you're shooting hoops.

349 BOULDER YOUR WAY TO BETTER ARMS

If rock climbing is perhaps just a bit too extreme for you but you'd love the upper-body benefits, then try the safer alternative of bouldering. This is a sport in which you travel along the rockface rather than scaling it upwards. It builds great arm strength and, as a bonus, burns a whopping 360 calories in just 30 minutes.

350 BOWL AWAY CALORIES

Next time you're playing a game of baseball, softball, rounders or cricket, volunteer to bowl or pitch – it burns the most calories of any other position on the playing field.

351 STEER CLEAR OF A CAFFEINE STITCH

To avoid a painful side stitch while you're exercising, avoid drinking caffeine for at least an hour before you start. Caffeine drinks, particularly if they are carbonated as well, have been shown to increase side-stitch pain.

352 PUNCH YOUR FIGHTS OUT

For the ultimate body- and brain-boosting workout, invest in a punchbag and a skipping rope. It has been shown that working out like a boxer will not only increase your cardiovascular fitness but also get rid of aggression and allow stress to flow out of the system.

353 WORKOUT BURNOUT

Overtraining can be just as dangerous as under-training. To prevent problems, make sure you have at least one complete rest day a week and give yourself a whole week off every two to three months to stay physically and mentally healthy.

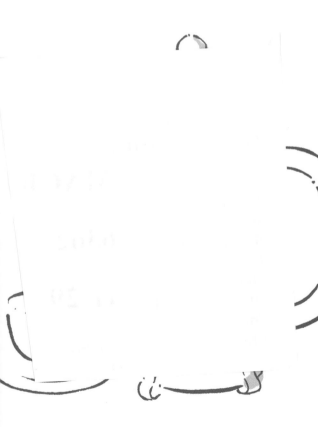

354 BANISH THE BANISTERS

Leaning on the banisters or handrail as you climb the stairs robs your legs of a strengthening workout. Keep your arms by your sides to boost strength and balance (and the same goes for the step machine).

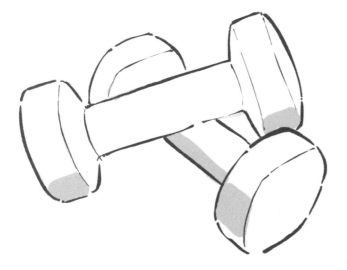

355 BOOST METABOLISM BY WORKING OUT EARLY

A workout first thing in the morning helps fire the metabolism all day, and when your metabolism is higher, you burn more calories. As a consequence, morning workouts mean you can eat the same amount and still lose weight.

356 BE STRETCH EFFECTIVE

Stretches are ineffective unless they are held for a certain time. You should ease into position until you feel the stretch, then hold it for at least 25 seconds. Breathe deeply to help your body move oxygen-rich blood to sore muscles.

357 GET RID OF YOUR JELLY BELLY

Belly dancing, because of its constant use of the abdominal and pelvic muscles, is one of the best exercises you can choose to tone up flabby bellies. It's fun, social and sexy, too – what more could you ask of a workout?

358 GO STRAIGHT FOR THE WEIGHTS

Experts suggest that weight training should be done before any cardiovascular work in the gym, because it requires fresh energy. Cardiovascular exercise requires less energy and helps flush toxins away from muscles, so it should be saved for the end of a workout session.

359 GET MORE FROM YOUR WORKOUT

During exercise that lasts more than 30 minutes, recent research shows that there is better performance, recovery and efficiency in people who drink at 10- to 20-minute intervals throughout the training session.

360 DON'T SIP UP

Sipping water little and often while you exercise isn't as effective at rehydrating your body as taking large gulps less often, because larger amounts of water travel through your stomach quicker and are more likely to be absorbed.

361 ASTHMA-FRIENDLY SPORTS

More than 10% of Olympic athletes suffer from asthma, so don't let it prevent you exercising. Go for sports near water, where asthma is less of a problem, like swimming, canoeing, sailing and windsurfing.

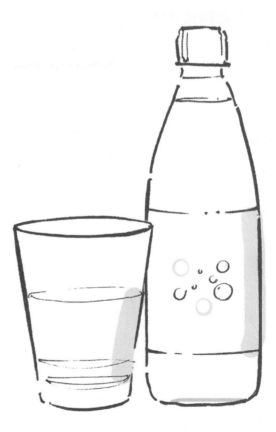

allergies

362 SMOKE GETS IN YOUR EYES

Keep rooms well ventilated. Fumes that hang in the air, such as those from fresh paint, tar fumes, air pollution, insect sprays and tobacco smoke, all aggravate allergic symptoms by irritating the sensitive mucous membranes in your eyes, nose and mouth.

363 STAY IN TO DRY OUT

To avoid windborne pollen and grass seeds coming into contact with you, sticking to your clothes and causing allergic reactions, dry clothes and bedding inside instead of hanging them out on a clothesline.

364 BRING BACK BATHTIME

Remember when the last thing you did before bed was have a bath? Washing your skin and hair in the evening rather than in the morning has been shown to reduce allergic reactions overnight by getting rid of allergens in hair and on skin.

365 HUNT FOR HIDDEN DAIRY

If milk doesn't agree with you and makes you sick, you need to be aware of products that contain hidden sources of some of the allergens it contains. Watch out for casein, sodium caseinate, lactoglobulin and nougat on ingredients labels.

366 IMAGINE YOURSELF SNEEZE-FREE

Studies have shown that, far from being quackery, taking some time out every day to think away your allergy could reap benefits. Take ten minutes in a quiet spot and create a mental image of yourself without your allergy – symptoms could begin to lessen after a few days.

367 A SWEET HEALER

The healing properties of honey are thought to flow from its high proportions of pollen and plant compounds, producing a natural immunity in the body. Bee pollen, royal jelly, honeycomb and unfiltered honey are all believed to help.

368 BREATHE NEW LIFE INTO YOUR THROAT

Mix up an inhalation mixture with hot water and a drop each of lavender, eucalyptus and camomile essential oils to soothe breathing and reduce swelling and inflammation of the nose and throat. To trap steam, cover your head with a towel and bend over to inhale.

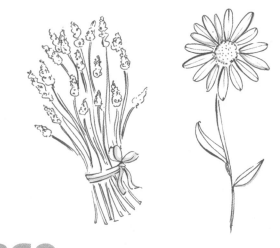

369 GO FOR GARLIC

Garlic is thought to boost immunity, which could help regulate the body's allergic reaction to pollen grains.

370 C FOR YOURSELF

Vitamin C is definitely the wonder vitamin when it comes to your immune system. Make sure you get a generous daily dose of fresh fruit and vegetables or take a supplement to keep your body fit to fight off infections.

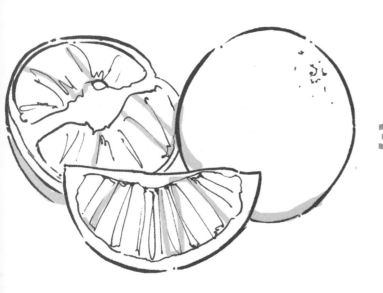

371 GET STEAMY TO CLEAR YOUR HEAD

Coughing during the night can be eased by hanging a wet towel on or near a radiator to increase humidity in the room overnight, preventing the lungs and throat from drying out and decreasing the chances of damage or infection.

372 GIVE IT SOME ELBOW GREASE

Some of the worst allergy irritants, such as formaldehyde, phenol and ammonia, are found in cleaning fluids. Think about using alternatives, such as vinegar, soda crystals, lemon juice, water and a bit of hard work!

373 DON'T STAND THE HEAT

A hot, humid house is a breeding ground for mould, mildew and dust mites. Turn down central heating to about 21°C (70°F) and if your house is humid, think about investing in an air-conditioning system or dehumidifier to help clear allergens.

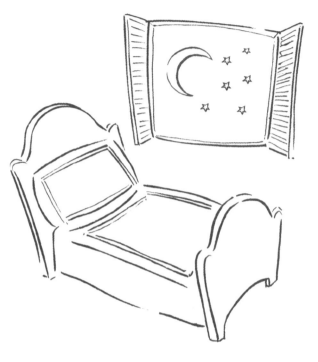

375 SOOTHE YOUR STRESS

Emotional stress can worsen responses to allergens, so relaxation techniques may help relieve the symptoms of allergic reaction, especially with breathing problems.

376 GET SALTY FOR SINUSES

If your sinuses are causing problems, you might want to try the 3,000-year-old yogic practice of sniffing saltwater, which can help fight and prevent sinus infections. Ask a doctor or nurse for advice.

arthritis

374 TREAT YOURSELF TO BREAKFAST IN BED

Habitual sneezing and coughing in the morning are often due to a sensitivity of the body to cold, so giving your body some time to get used to the temperature change first thing by eating a warm breakfast or drink in bed could help prevent these irritants.

377 GO ALKALINE TO NEUTRALIZE ACID PAIN

Acidic foods like tomato, citrus fruits, fruit juices and red meats can make the pain of arthritis worse by building up acid crystals in the joints. Instead, plump for high-alkaline or neutral foods like green vegetables, eggs, dairy produce and water.

91

378 EASE PAIN WITH PINEAPPLE

Pineapple has been shown to suppress inflammation and boost bone health, thus improving joint pain in arthritis. Its anti-inflammatory properties are thought to be due to its high bromelain content.

379 BOTH HANDS FOR LIGHT LIFTING

Using both of your hands rather than just one when lifting frying pans, pouring water from a kettle or jug, and carrying heavy household items eases the stress and strain that is caused by friction on joints and it can as a result reduce the effects of pain and discomfort.

380 GET A JELLY GOOD CURE

A daily supplement containing gelatine, which has unique physical and chemical properties that enable it to reverse the effects of arthritis, can help ease arthritis symptoms significantly after three months of taking it.

381 STEER CLEAR OF SAUCES

Condiments and sauces like mustard, mayonnaise and vinegar can disrupt the pH of the body, turning it acidic and causing more pain to arthritic joints. Use natural yogurt as a garnish or opt for tomato-based sauces.

382 GO LARGE FOR A BETTER GRIP

If you suffer from the problems associated with arthritis of the hands, life in the kitchen will be far easier if you choose gadgets and equipment fitted with large handles. Alternatively, wrap tape or foam around skinny handles so they are easier on your hands when you grip them.

383 LEVER YOURSELF TO FREEDOM

If you have a weak grip, rather than struggling with hard-to-turn taps (faucets), why not fit levers? These will make your life much easier, as you will have to exert far less strength to turn them on and off. You could also replace doorknobs with levers to help you with doors.

384 SOAK AWAY PAIN

Morning baths in warm water, or soaks for feet and hands, can help ease pain from arthritic joints, which is often worse first thing. Soak for at least ten minutes to reap maximum benefits.

385 GO ELECTRIC FOR TIP-TOP TEETH

An electric toothbrush makes it easier to maintain dental health despite difficulty gripping with arthritic hand joints.

386 TAKE UP TAI CHI FOR FLEXIBILITY

The ancient Chinese art of Tai Chi has been shown to reduce both the effects of arthritis and the distress caused by stiff, painful joints. Practising at least two or three times a week is most beneficial.

387 STEP OUT AND STRETCH OUT

Regular walking, light weightlifting and stretching can reduce the pain from arthritis by up to a third. Aim for 20–30 minutes of exercise every day and mix it up for maximum pain relief.

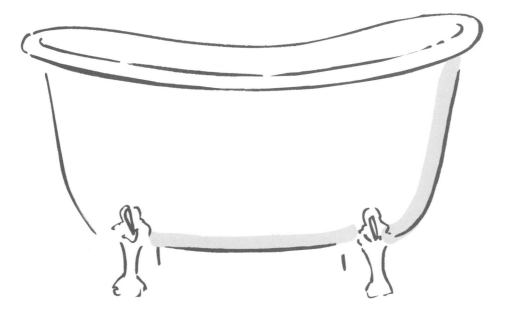

388 CURRY FLAVOUR TO STOP SWELLING

Curries that contain high levels of the herb turmeric contain circumin, a natural anti-inflammatory that can help alleviate pain and swelling. If you don't fancy the hot stuff, supplements are also available.

389 DROP A SIZE TO BE KNEE-WISE

According to experts, being overweight is such a danger to joints that losing as little as 5kg (11lb) may cut the risk of osteoarthritis of the knee by 50%.

390 RUE THE RHUBARB

Rhubarb contains oxalic acid, which inhibits your body's ability to absorb calcium and iron from other foods. It can aggravate arthritis and may even cause an attack if eaten to excess.

391 BE SUPER-CAREFUL IN THE SUN

Arthritis can make the skin more sensitive to the sun, so make sure you cover head, shoulders and eyes on bright days.

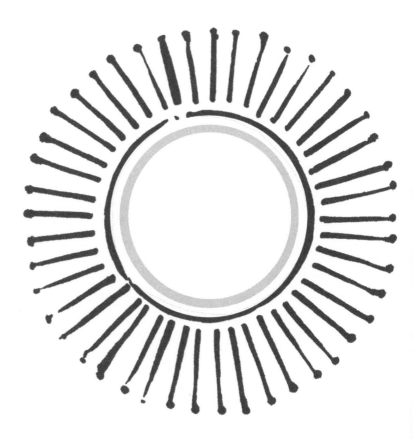

back pain

392 DESTRESS TO HELP YOUR BACK

Stress causes muscle tension that can lead to pain, especially in the lower back as the postural support muscles are overworked. Experts estimate that almost a fifth of all back pain is due to stress, so relaxation could be the most important prevention.

393 HAIL A TAXI TO HEAD OFF INJURY

Choosing comfortable shoes, with a small heel to support the feet, could be key to back health. Each 2.5cm (1in) on the heel doubles the strain on joints and can throw the pelvis off balance, so avoid walking too far in them on those glamorous nights out.

394 QUICK-RELEASE YOUR BACK

For a quick back stretch at your desk, place your feet flat on the ground and lean back on your chair so your back arches slightly. Drop your head backwards and then take a few deep breaths.

395 DON'T BE AN ARCH VILLAIN

The spine begins to show signs of wear and tear as early as age 35, so from this age onwards it's important to keep it flexible and strong. Lots of people forget that the back doesn't only bend forward – it's important to stretch it into an arched position as well. You can do this by simply leaning backwards to release muscles or try backwards bend yoga postures.

396 BEND INTO GOOD POSTURE

Many back problems are caused by adopting a bad lifting posture and by carrying heavy objects incorrectly. The best lifting posture is where the legs, not the back, do the work. So, when lifting, be certain to bend the knees and always carry heavy objects close to the body at waist level.

397 BAG A HEALTHY BACK

Carrying your bag on the same shoulder all the time can lead to muscle imbalance and weakness, leading to pain. Resolve to swap shoulders every other day or use a backpack.

398 BED DOWN IN COMFORT

Sleeping on your stomach can put the back and neck into various strained positions, causing stiffness and pain when you wake in the morning. To prevent problems developing, lie flat on your back with a pillow under your knees. Or sleep on your side with knees slightly bent and a pillow between your legs.

399 LOSE WEIGHT TO LESSEN PAIN

Being overweight forces your body to carry more than its natural weight and, as most people walk at least a mile every day just in normal life, every pound counts. Slimming down could help most overweight people with back problems.

400 GO HOT AND COLD TO STOP SWELLING

Using cold packs for five to ten minutes at a time on affected areas will reduce inflammation. If the pain lingers after 24 hours, switch to heat treatment with hot towels or a shower or bath.

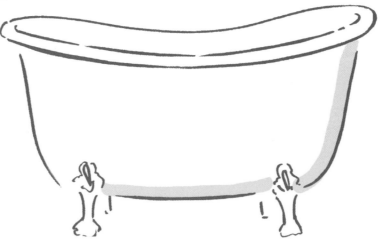

401 DON'T STOP MOVING

Studies show that people with acute back pain who go about their everyday activities as normally as possible heal better than those who rest, because movement naturally causes the body to pump fluid into the spongy discs that separate and cushion the vertebrae in your back. So don't rest too much unless you have to.

402 SIT UP WITH SIT-UPS

It is estimated that strengthening the abdominal muscles could prevent more than 75% of lower-back problems. Regular sit-ups and abdominal exercises can help, as can core strength training with Pilates and yoga classes.

403 GIVE YOUR BACK SOME BACK-UP

Use a chair with a proper backrest to prevent pressure on the lower back, or slip a thin cushion or rolled-up jumper (sweater) behind your lower back for correct support.

404 BE A SCREEN SIREN

Make sure your computer screen is at the right height for comfortable viewing – you shouldn't need to lean towards or away from your screen, for example, and it should be level with your eyes. In addition, your arms should rest lightly on the desk's surface as you use the keyboard.

405 IT'S HIP TO STRETCH

Many back problems stem from the hips. Stretch out your hip flexor muscles by lying on the floor with one leg flat and the other bent at the knee. Then slowly pull the bent leg towards your chest while pressing your whole back to the floor. Hold this position for 30 seconds.

406 SITTING PRETTY

When sitting at a desk for long periods of time, rest your feet flat on the floor or use a foot support to prevent the weight of the lower legs being supported by the front of the thighs.

407 STRAIGHTEN THOSE LEGS

Bear in mind that you shouldn't cross your legs, which can cause the pelvis and hips to tilt and strain, or have your thighs pressing against your chair seat too firmly, as this puts pressure on the veins on the underside of your thighs.

408 HAVE A SIESTA FOR PRESSURE-FREE EVENINGS

The pressure on the back is more than two and a half times greater when sitting than when you are standing, and a massive ten times greater when you are sitting rather than lying down. In light of this, a ten-minute nap or lie-down in the afternoon could deliver enormous back benefits.

409 QUIT SMOKING FOR HEALTHIER SPINAL DISCS

Smokers are more likely to suffer back pain that non-smokers because nicotine restricts the flow of blood to the intervertebral discs that cushion the spine.

410 MAKE LIKE A CAT TO STRETCH YOUR BACK

To ease the strain and any discomfort in your back, get down on your hands and knees, hands palm down in line with shoulders, looking at the floor. Slowly push your back up into an upward curve, hold this for five seconds and then release. Repeat this ten times.

411 DON'T EVEN THINK ABOUT IT

It would now appear that the old wives' tale is right after all – the more you think about your pain, the worse it will feel. Researchers have found that the people who don't pay any attention to their pain seem to suffer less.

412 SWIM INTO HEALTH

Swimming is an excellent exercise for healthy backs because it avoids the strain of impact sports and allows the body to realign itself while supported by the water.

413 TILT YOUR PELVIS TO TREAT YOUR BACK

Try this pelvic exercise to ease any stress you might be feeling in the lower back region. Lie flat on your back with your legs bent and feet flat on the floor. Press your lower back to the floor by tightening the abdominal muscles; hold for ten seconds and then release the position. Repeat five times, breathing normally throughout.

414 PACK SOME HEAT TO DULL PAIN

To relieve chronic pain and stiffness in your back, try heated water therapies such as swimming pools, whirlpools, warm showers and steam rooms. Alternatively, apply warm compresses, hot towels or microwaveable heat packs to the area.

415 TOP UP ON CALCIUM

Calcium is essential for keeping the bones of the spine firm and flexible. There are plenty of sources besides milk, including yogurt, broccoli, kale, figs, almonds and calcium supplements.

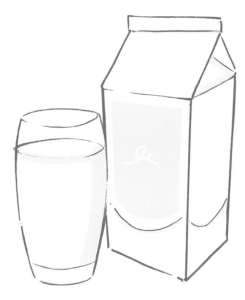

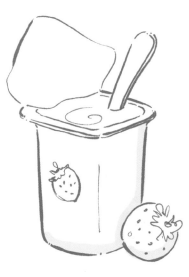

416 CURTAIL YOUR CAFFEINE

While you may be convinced that you really need the extra burst of energy that coffee provides in the morning, try to resist the temptation to have those second and third cups. Recent studies show that the extra caffeine can actually weaken bones.

beating cancer

417 AWARE IT WELL

Being aware of changes in your body is a surefire way to catch cancer early, boosting chances of effective treatment. Know how your skin looks and feels to track changes.

418 SWEAT IT AWAY

Studies have shown that regular physical exercise prompts a series of changes within the body that actively fight cancer. The risk of colon, breast, prostate and other cancers lessens with regular activity.

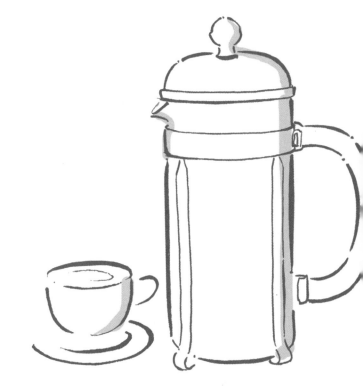

418 A GREAT WHEY TO BEAT BREAST CANCER

Whey – this is the watery part of milk that remains when the curds have been separated – could help protect against breast cancer by reducing the hormone oestrogen. Experts also believe that soy sauce could have a similar effect.

420 SPROUT A DOUBLE CANCER CURE

Green leafy vegetables contain a combination of two components that are 13 times more powerful at fighting cancer together than alone. Selenium and sulphoraphane are found in high levels in Brussels sprouts, broccoli and cabbage.

421 COUNT CALCIUM TO FIGHT CANCER

Low-fat diets that limit intake of dairy products could be exposing slimmers to colon cancer by reducing their calcium intake to dangerously low levels. Studies suggest that even small increases in calcium can cut the risk by half.

422 GET A PIZZA FOR ANTICANCER ACTION

Pizzas aren't all bad, and the more tomato sauce they have on top, the better. The powerful antioxidant lycopene, which makes tomatoes red, has protective effects against cancer. Cooked tomatoes are best.

423 GO GREEN TO PROTECT YOURSELF

The polyphenols and catechins in green tea have powerful antioxidative and anticancer effects when taken regularly. Aim for at least one cup a day.

424 VEG OUT ON FRUIT

Fresh fruit and vegetables are such powerful anticancer agents that they can even lower the risk of lung cancer in heavy smokers.

425 PEACHY KEEN

Peaches, sweet potatoes and apricots contain high levels of betacarotene, which cannot only prevent cancer cells from growing but can even kill them off.

426 BE A LEMON TO FIGHT DISEASE

Citrus fruits, such as grapefruit, lemon and orange, are powerful anticancer agents because they contain a collection of all the natural substances known to ward off cancer cells.

427 GET SMELLY TO GET HEALTHY

Pungent foods like onion and garlic not only have a powerful effect on cancer tumours but also work to boost the function of the immune system.

428 UNDERCOOK FOR GOOD HEALTH

Charring food during roasting, grilling and barbecueing can produce carcinogens in the burned areas. The healthiest food is cooked through but not burned.

429 SPOON OUT SPINACH

Spinach contains gluthione, a powerful anticancer agent. Gluthione is found in lower levels in other green leafy vegetables, too.

430 EAT UP A RAINBOW

Everyone seems to recognize that the red-coloured fruits and vegetables are good for us, but don't forget your other colours, too. For example, a low intake of green- and yellow-coloured vegetables has been linked to the development of cervical and breast cancers.

431 BE A GOOD BEAN

Eating beans, including chickpeas, kidney beans and lentils, on a regular basis – say, one portion every week – could cut the risk of death from cancer by nearly half. This is because beans contain various anticancer agents.

432 TRAIN YOUR TASTEBUDS

Sugar is a major risk factor for cancer. Instead of choosing high-sugar options, train your tastebuds by gradually reducing sugar in your diet or swapping it for healthy alternatives, such as apple juice, date sugar and rice syrup.

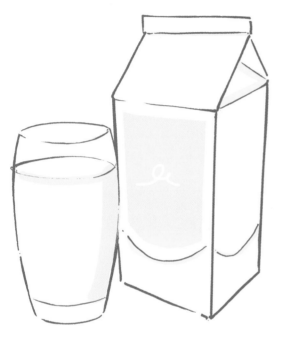

434 PICK YOUR WAY TO A CURE

Blackberries and raspberries are great anticancer agents because of their high levels of antioxidants. The fresher the better, so pick your own for best results.

435 KEEP IT FRESH

Aflatoxins, thought to be linked to liver cancers, can develop in peanuts, corn and pepper when stored for a long time. If in doubt, use only fresh ingredients.

436 CRESS YOUR ANTICANCER BUTTONS

Watercress contains a cancer-fighting substance called phenethyl isothiocyanate, thought to act against tumours, particularly in lung cancer.

433 MILK PROTECTS YOUR BELLY

Large quantities of high-fat milk have been shown to increase chances of bowel and colon cancer, but low-fat milk can actually protect the digestive system from disease.

437 DON'T GET IN A PICKLE

Some pickles, dried meats and fish contain high levels of preservative nitrites, and these may be linked to stomach cancer. Try making your own chutneys or look closely at labels to see what has been included.

breathing problems

438 TALK THE TALK

A good way to keep your breathing calm and regular is to have a conversation with someone or to read out loud. Speech naturally regulates breathing, thus putting a stop to the short and shallow breaths that can lead to problems.

439 BREATHE NATURALLY

More than a fifth of all adults with asthma have some sensitivity to aspirin, and many also have problems with other painkillers such as ibuprofen. Be careful what you take if you have breathing problems.

440 TAKE A DEEP BREATH

Taking a few deep breaths really does help you stay calm and in control, by stopping the release of the stress hormones adrenaline and cortisol into the blood.

441 DON'T SAY LOW, SAY NO

Studies reveal that the risk of contracting lung cancer is no different in people who smoke medium-tar cigarettes, low-tar cigarettes or very low-tar cigarettes, so instead of opting for a low-tar version of your favourite brand, experts recommend that giving up entirely is the only way to protect your lungs.

442 STRIKE A POSE

Yoga has been shown to help breathing problems and asthma by reducing tension in the breathing muscles and expanding the ribs to allow more air inside the lungs. Aim for three sessions a week to reap the health rewards.

443 BREATHE EASY WITH BUTEYKO

The Buteyko technique – a method of breathing correction and concentration – has been found to reduce and cure asthma in even serious cases. Ask your doctor for advice or visit www.buteyko.com.

444 VITALIZE LUNGS WITH VITAMINS

A lack of vitamins C and E, betacarotene and selenium (found in lentils, avocados and brazil nuts) in the diet can harm the lungs so much that it's the equivalent of smoking a pack of 20 cigarettes a day for ten years.

445 EAT ONION TO PREVENT CANCER

Eating lots of onion, apple and yellow grapefruit regularly could help protect your body against developing lung cancer by destroying squamous cell carcinoma, which is a specific type of the disease. Combine cooked onion with raw apple and grapefruit for the most potent anticancer effect.

446 POOL YOUR RESOURCES

Swimming is the no. 1 activity for healthy lungs because they're forced to work to their optimal potential as you exercise and restrict breathing. But you've got to put your head underwater to benefit.

colds & flu

447 LISTEN TO YOUR ELDERS

Elderberry flowers contain flavonoids and tannins, substances that reduce fever and promote sweating. The berries are rich in vitamin C, which may prevent flu infection, while other compounds bind to the flu virus and prevent it from penetrating cell walls.

448 THINK ZINC FOR SORE THROATS

Zinc gluconate lozenges may shorten colds by an average of three days as well as alleviate sore throats, nasal congestion, coughing, headaches and hoarseness.

449 TAKE A BREAK IF YOU'RE FEELING LOW

Extreme amounts of exercise increase the body's production of harmful free radicals, which heighten your risk of succumbing to colds and viruses and can generally cause you to feel run down.

450 DON'T OVERLOAD ON WATER

Many people's first reaction when they come down with a respiratory infection is to drink copious amounts of water. However, some experts now believe that overdrinking could worsen the problem by leading to salt loss and fluid overload. Aim for 2 litres (3½ pints) a day.

451 CHEERS FOR IMMUNITY

Experts believe wine could be a powerful ally against the common cold by boosting immunity to the hundreds of viruses that cause it. Studies have found that people who drink moderately have a lower risk of catching colds.

452 WASH AWAY GERMS

Cold and flu viruses access your body through broken skin or the mucous membranes in your eyes and nose. Most people touch their face without realizing it, so wash your hands regularly to avoid passing on the virus.

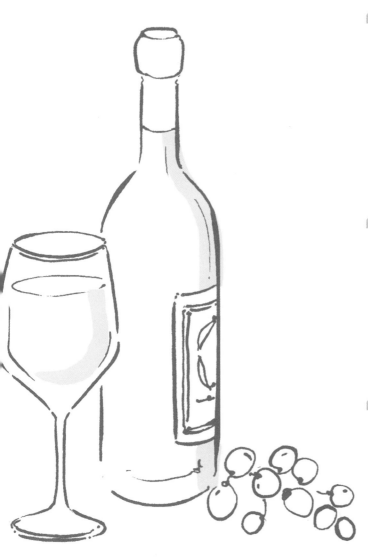

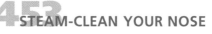

453 STEAM-CLEAN YOUR NOSE

The steam from boiling water can help your system fight off infections, possibly by killing any viruses that have newly alighted in the mucous membranes of your nose. To stay healthy, get down to your local sauna or steam room or invest in a facial steamer for home use.

454 GET BY WITH A LITTLE HELP FROM YOUR FRIENDS

Studies show that the more friends you have, the less likely you are to succumb to a cold. This is because you will handle stress better, making you less likely to fall foul of viruses.

455 STOP GARGLING TO HELP YOUR SORE THROAT

Gargling when you've got a sore throat is the equivalent of rubbing your eyes when they're sore. Instead, drink soothing warm – but not hot – liquids with a spoonful of honey to help your throat heal.

456 CUT PAINKILLERS FOR AN EARLY CURE

If you can handle it, cutting back on taking painkillers regularly when you have a cold may help you recover a day earlier by allowing the virus to run its course.

457 STICK YOUR TONGUE OUT AT COLDS

Pour hot water into a bowl and breathe in, sticking your tongue out as you do so. This opens the throat and allows more steam through to prevent membranes drying out.

458 SCHEDULE SOME SHUT-EYE

Sleeping helps your body as well as your brain, so give your immune system a helping hand in virus season by aiming to sleep for seven to eight hours a night.

459 SNIFF AWAY SYMPTOMS

Aromatherapy oils of black pepper, eucalyptus, hyssop, pine and sweet thyme can help get rid of coughs, colds and symptoms of congestion. Use with steam to alleviate symptoms further.

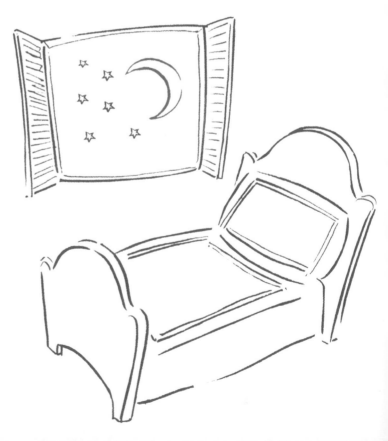

460 MAKE TIME FOR TEA

Regular tea drinking could boost your immune system. Black, green and oolong teas all contain the bacteria-fighting chemical L-theanine, which can protect against colds.

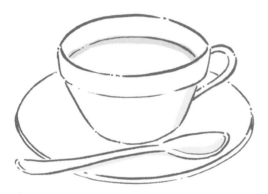

461 AVOID THE FALLOUT

A sneeze can travel at 160kph (100mph) and is a very common way for colds and flu to spread. Look for the telltale warning signs of an erupting sneeze and make sure you get out of the way of the spray.

462 SOUP IT UP

Chicken soup helps the cilia (tiny hairs) of the nose and bronchial passages move quickly so they can defend the respiratory system against contagions, and it contains substances that help the immune system fight off attack.

fever

463 COVER UP IN MODERATION

If you have a fever, don't cover up under too many blankets or take a hot shower, which may raise your temperature higher. Instead, try to keep to a normal covering.

464 KNOW YOUR BODY'S LIMITS

Normal body temperature is 37°C (98.6°F). Contact your doctor for temperatures above 38.5°C (101°F) that last more than a day and seek emergency attention for temperatures of 40°C (104°F) or more.

465 DON'T OD ON VITAMIN C

When you get a fever, the tendency is to reach for vitamin C, but be careful not to go overboard. Too much can lead to diarrhoea and kidney stones.

466 SPURN PILLS FOR SPEEDY RECOVERY

Lowering temperatures with drugs might help in the short term but research has shown that the body may recover better if mild temperatures are left untreated.

467 CUT OUT MEAT TO CUT THE HEAT

Reducing iron if you have a temperature could help fight infection, so avoid iron-rich foods until you're on the mend, then stock up your levels as you recover.

468 MAKE YOUR TEMPERATURE TEPID

To ease the discomfort of a fever, don't use cold water, which can shock the skin into holding onto heat. Instead, get into a bath that feels the same as body temperature or dab yourself with a tepid flannel.

first aid

468 LAVENDER CURES

Lavender oil works well on cuts, wounds, dermatitis, eczema, nappy (diaper) rash, pimples, insect bites and burns, while lavender or camomile essential oils can be added to a bath to soothe minor sunburn.

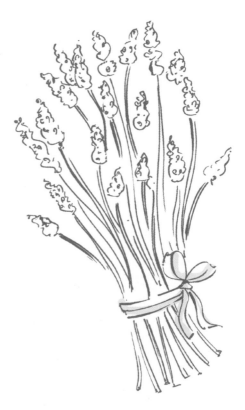

470 BE INFECTION-FREE WITH TEA TREE

Cleansing, antiseptic tea tree oil can be applied directly to skin in order to help keep minor scrapes and wounds clean, and it has been shown to be a more powerful antibiotic than many modern drugs. Keep some handy in your medicine cabinet for day-to-day use.

471 DON'T GET STUNG WITH AFTER-PAIN

If you are stung by a bee, carefully grasp and pull out the stinger as fast as you can. The less venom that enters your body, the smaller and less painful the resulting welt will be. Ice the area immediately to reduce the swelling.

472 A NATURAL ALTERNATIVE TO ANTIBIOTICS

Eucalyptus oil has long been prized for its healing abilities, but recent research studies have shown that it can be even more effective at fighting bacterial infections than some antibiotics.

473 TELL THE TOOTH ABOUT MILK

Teeth that have been knocked out, perhaps in a sporting activity or as the result of a fight or accident, can be successfully replanted up to 24 hours later – but only if the teeth have been stored in whole milk. Drop the teeth immediately into some cold whole milk and get to a dentist as soon as you possibly can.

474 LEAN FORWARDS FOR NOSEBLEEDS

For nosebleeds, the age-old remedy of tilting the head back can actually increase blood flow. Instead, tilt the head slightly forward and pinch the soft part of the nose. When the bleeding stops, don't blow your nose for at least four hours.

475 DON'T FEEL THE BURN

Douse minor burns immediately with cold water for at least ten minutes. Cover major burns with clingfilm (plastic wrap), apply cold water or ice over the top and call for medical attention at once.

476 KEEP BERRY COOL

On hot summer days, when heatstroke is a possible hazard, enhance the body's natural cooling system with infusions of raspberry and peppermint tea.

477 FIGHT BITES WITH CITRONELLA

The aromas of tea tree, eucalyptus and citronella have been shown to repel mosquitoes and other biting insects, so apply the oils to exposed areas of the skin to ensure you don't get bitten.

478 SAY ALOE TO CALMER SKIN

Aloe vera has soothing properties that stop the inflammation and redness of skin rashes, including prickly heat. Apply liberally for best results.

479 SOOTHE SPOTS WITH CALENDULA

Calendula oil or ointment is another great helper for skin problems. It soothes and draws out heat, making it useful for bites, stings, blisters and other skin ailments.

headaches

480 TRY TEMPLE MASSAGE

Massaging the temples in a circular motion with aromatherapy oils helps ease the pain of migraine and tension headaches, as well as reducing stuffiness and eye pain.

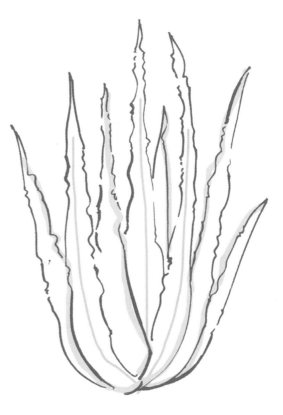

481 HOOK A HEADACHE CURE

Omega-3 essential fatty acids (EFAs), found in oily fish such as tuna and salmon, can lower the production of hormones that cause inflammation and pain, so eating fish regularly could help stop those migraines once and for all.

482 PUT JAW PAIN IN LINE

Many headaches are due to stress and tension in the muscles of the jaw. Check if your jaw might be to blame by sitting in front of a mirror and opening and closing your mouth slowly in a straight line. Many people find that their jaws are way off line at the beginning of the exercise.

483 WATER DOWN THE TENDERNESS

Give yourself a pain-relieving massage by standing in the shower with the water stream directed to the back of your neck, then slowly turning to look behind you. This removes lactic acid from the muscles and makes the blood vessels less 'irritable'.

484 FEAST ON FEVERFEW

Feverfew contains niacin (a B vitamin) and iron, and provides nutrition to the central nervous system and alleviates migraines. At the onset of a headache, try a sandwich of feverfew leaves or brew up a warm tea.

485 PAIN BETWEEN THE EYES

Less than perfect eyesight can trigger headaches because the eye and other muscles squeeze in order to focus. If your headaches come on after reading or working at a computer screen, make sure you give your eyes a rest every ten minutes by focusing on a distant object for at least 60 seconds. Make a point of having regular eye examinations, too.

486 AVOID THE HOT AND COLD OF IT

Extreme chilling or warming of the neck can bring on headaches by altering blood flow to the head, which replicates the migraine mechanism. Wear a scarf if you're moving between different temperatures.

487 PILL YOURSELF TOGETHER

Headache sufferers who take lots of pain-killers could be giving themselves more pain with rebound headaches as they withdraw from their regular dose. If you think this might be you, see your doctor.

488 CHANGE YOUR BRA TO CURE YOUR HEAD

Overtight bra straps can dig into the shoulder and put pressure on the cervical nerve, causing frequent headaches. Full-breasted women are most likely to suffer from this, but all women are at risk. Buy bras with wide straps and check that your bra fits correctly around the chest.

489 INDULGE IN A SPOT OF COFFEE THERAPY

Coffee can help cure headaches because of the injection of caffeine it gives the body (but take care not to overdo the caffeine – many over-the-counter headache remedies already contain a healing dose).

490 GO BANANAS

If your headaches tend to come on in the late mornings, late afternoons or after a long lie-in, they might be due to low blood sugar (hypoglycaemia). These headaches can be helped by eating foods that release sugar slowly, such as bananas, wholegrains and oats.

491 HOLD THE HOT DOGS

Some people are very sensitive to the nitrites that are used as a preservative in a range of processed meats, especially hot dogs, burgers and cold cuts. Avoid these foods and, if your headaches disappear, stay off them.

492 SNIFF AN APPLE A DAY

Apples could keep the doctor away after all. Research studies have shown that the scent of green apples can reduce the severity of migraines, so the next time you feel a headache coming on, reach for the fruit bowl and inhale deeply.

493 BITE THE BULLET

Poor tooth or jaw alignment has been found to be the cause of some chronic headaches. A few sessions in the dentist's chair could clear your head for good.

494 COME DOWN FROM ON HIGH

Headaches that usually occur only when you're angry, during vigorous exercise, and/or right before sexual orgasm could be down to high blood pressure, especially if accompanied by redness or throbbing. See your doctor if this sounds familiar.

heart disease

495 GIVE YOURSELF A PERFECT TEN

It's just about safe to be 4.5kg (10lb) too heavy, but no more than this, according to heart experts, who have found that even an excess of 5kg (11lb) can significantly increase the risk of heart disease.

496 EGGS ON THE MENU AGAIN

Eggs contain heart-protective nutrients including antioxidants, folate, other B vitamins and unsaturated fat that can counteract the effects of saturated fat and cholesterol.

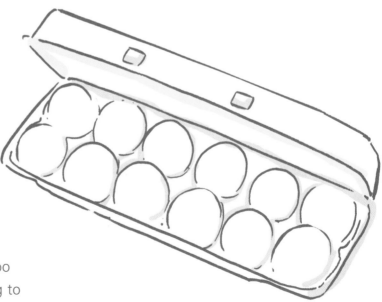

497 NUTS FOR A HEALTHY HEART

Nuts are rich in unsaturated fats and vitamin E, which have been linked to a reduced risk of heart disease in nut eaters, who are a third less likely to suffer such problems than other people.

498 SAY ALOE TO A HEALTHY HEART

A diet that is supplemented with aloe vera and psyllium husks could set you on the road to having better heart health by reducing the amount of cholesterol in your system and improving the balance of good and bad cholesterol.

499 GIVE ME MORE THAN FIVE

Don't stop at the recommended five portions of fruit and vegetables every day. Eating more could give you an extra health boost, with every additional serving estimated to lower the risk of heart disease by 4%. One serving is an apple or orange, a large spoonful of vegetables or a handful of grapes, cherries or chopped fruit.

500 GET HEARTY WITH VITAMIN E

Acting as a mild anticoagulant, vitamin E reduces the risk of blood clots and the oxidation of cholesterol, inhibiting production of fatty deposits that can block blood vessels and cause the onset of heart problems.

501 GARLIC BREATH IS HEALTHY BREATH

Garlic and onions, along with other members of the onion family like leeks and chives, have been shown to halve the risk of cancer if eaten regularly.

502 EARN SOME FAT PROFITS

Not all fat is bad. Beneficial essential fatty acids (EFAs), such as the omega-3 type found in fish, olives and flaxseed, have been shown to reduce the risk of heart disease. Instead of banning fat entirely from your diet, substitute good fats for the heart-harming trans fats found in many margarines, cooking oils and processed foods.

503 STEER CLEAR OF HYDROGENATED OILS

Just a few grams of omega-3 fatty acids a day can prevent an irregular heart beat, decrease inflammation and promote blood flow. Choose olive oil and fish oils instead of cooking oils, because the hydrogenation process they go through destroys omega-3.

joint problems

504 GET OFF YOUR HIGH HEELS

Heels force the thigh muscles to work harder, putting extra strain on the knee joint and tendons, so if you want bunion-free, perfect feet, it's best to go flat.

505 KEEP IT SLOW TO REMAIN PAIN-FREE

Muscles adapt quickly to new exercises or movements, but joints, ligaments and tendons take longer. Ease yourself into new activities over a course of weeks or months to avoid the risk of injury.

506 SOOTHE PAIN WITH GINGER

In a recent trial, 63% of patients taking ginger reported a reduction in knee pain while standing, compared with 50% of those who took the placebo. Those taking ginger also reported less pain after walking a distance of 15m (50ft).

507 OIL YOUR JOINTS WITH BORAGE

Arthritis sufferers who have pain, joint tenderness, swelling and soreness, particularly first thing in the morning, could relieve their symptoms significantly by taking borage-oil capsules, a supplement made from the garden herb.

508 GIVE BONES A D-DAY

Calcium isn't all we need to keep bones healthy and strong and guard against osteoporosis as we get older. Studies have shown that vitamin D in association with calcium boosts the body's ability to make the most of both substances to increase bone health and strength.

509 WARM UP TO AVOID INJURY

Gently warming up your body before undertaking an exercise routine can be likened to warming your car up on a winter's morning before setting off. To keep your body running smoothly, start the session slowly and get up to speed only after your muscles and joints have had at least five minutes of preparation.

510 OPT FOR OLIVES FOR HEALTHY JOINTS

People who eat the most olive oil and cooked vegetables are about 75% less likely to develop rheumatoid arthritis than those who eat the fewest servings, so don't beat yourself up about having that extra oil.

511 GET WITH THE PROGRAMME

Exercise reduces pain. In one study, patients with osteoarthritis of the knee were able to reduce the amount of pain medication they took after participating in an eight-week walking programme.

512 GALVANIZE SORE JOINTS WITH GLUCOSAMINE

Truly the wonder drug where the body's joints are concerned, glucosamine occurs naturally in the body. In studies it has been shown, time after time, to strengthen joints, reduce pain, prevent injury and help protect against the degeneration that comes with ageing. Glucosamine is even more effective when taken with chondroitin, a closely related substance that prevents body enzymes from degrading joint cartilage.

513 STEP OUT TO EASE STIFFNESS

Exercise, tailored to the individual's abilities, is well known to ease joint stiffness. People suffering from rheumatoid arthritis have cut the amount of time they feel stiff each morning by an average of 68 minutes after just six weeks of regular exercise and physical therapy. Physical exercise actually combats fatigue and sufferers report that they feel less tired after they begin a regular exercise programme.

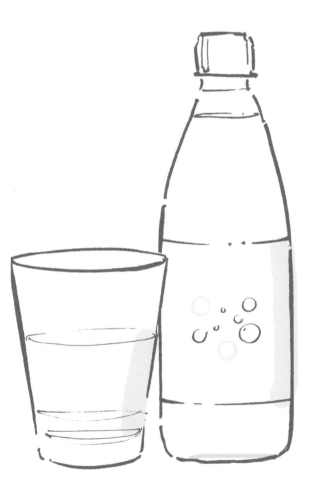

muscle soreness

514 DRINK UP TO STOP STIFFNESS

Dehydration is a major cause of post-exercise muscle soreness. Drinking water regularly while you work out should be sufficient to keep levels high enough to combat pain.

515 REDUCE PAIN WITH VITAMIN C

Vitamin C and bioflavonoids may help offset the damage that muscles endure during exercise. Taken regularly, these nutrients reduce the incidence of sports injuries and shorten the time it takes to recover from a muscle injury.

516 WISE UP TO WARMING UP

Prepare yourself for your workout by moving a little first to get the blood flowing. This will help supply the muscles with oxygenated blood, which will prevent injuries and reduce lactic acid buildup in muscle fibres.

517 A PINEAPPLE PICK-UP

Bromelain, which is a fruit extract taken from the pineapple, has potent anti-inflammatory properties in the body that can help to reduce muscle soreness brought about by inflammation. And the fruit gives you a good dose of vitamins that help healing, too.

518 STROKE AWAY SORENESS

Massage can help reduce the pain that results from overexercised muscles by stimulating the blood flow in the affected areas, helping lymphatic drainage and promoting tissue repair. Visit a sports masseur or do it yourself with long, gentle strokes towards the heart.

519 BUILD UP SLOWLY

The greatest incidence of muscle soreness happens in untrained people. Avoid this by gradually increasing exercise intensity over five or six sessions so the untrained muscles can progressively adapt.

520 STAY PAIN-FREE WITH VITAMIN E

Recent research studies have shown that taking daily vitamin E supplements helps reduce muscle soreness when taken for at least a week before a strenuous exercise session. Get your daily dose naturally from vitamin-rich fruit and vegetables, or take a vitamin supplement.

521 WIND DOWN SLOWLY

Warm down for a few minutes after strenuous exercise sessions, lowering your heart rate gradually back to its normal level with a low-intensity routine. Cool down after every workout with long, static stretches.

522 REMEMBER THE RICE RULE

RICE stands for rest, ice, compression and elevation, and is a great way to reduce soreness. Rest allows healing, ice and compression stave off inflammation and bruising, and elevation (raising the affected area above the heart) drains excess fluid.

523 DRINK SMOOTHIES TO HEAL MUSCLE TEARS

Combine calcium-rich milk with potassium-packed banana for a smoothie to treat muscles cramps and soreness after exercise. Calcium and potassium help muscles heal microtears that can cause pain.

526 CRUNCH ON CRACKERS

Eat high-carbohydrate foods such as dry crackers and toast if you're troubled by nausea. They move through the stomach quickly and may be helpful if eaten soon after you wake up in the morning.

nausea

524 ROOT OUT SICKNESS

Ginger root, taken as powder or tea, works directly in the gastrointestinal tract by interfering with the feedback mechanisms that send sickness messages to the brain.

525 PRESS AWAY DISCOMFORT

Acupressure wrist bands, which attach around the forearm and press against certain antisickness acupressure points, have been shown to help prevent motion sickness and nausea.

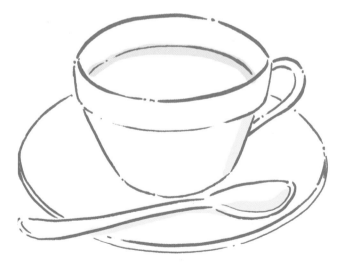

527 INFUSE AN ANTISICKNESS TEA

Catnip, raspberry leaf, mint, fennel and, of course, ginger, all make great herbal infusions to help prevent nausea and sickness. Check the labels carefully if you are using them to treat morning sickness, however, as raspberry leaf should be avoided in early pregnancy.

528 OUT OF THE KITCHEN

If food smells nauseate you, stay out of the kitchen while meals are prepared – even leave the house, if necessary. Cold foods tend to have less odour, so try eating chicken or salad sandwiches, chilled soups, yogurt and fruit.

529 CHEW IT OVER

Nausea can be caused by indigestion, but this can be prevented by adequate chewing of food. Many people gulp down food in large lumps; these are difficult to digest and so can cause trapped wind and general gut discomfort.

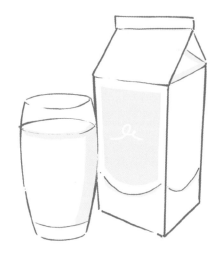

530 BE WARY OF DAIRY

With the exception of yogurt, dairy products should be avoided if you've been vomiting until the problem is quite resolved. Orange juice, grapefruit juice and fried, spicy or fatty foods should also be avoided completely in favour of dry foods and plain water.

531 BECOME AN OLD SOAK

Soaking beans in water can help turn their indigestible, wind- and nausea-inducing components into easier-to-digest substances. For the best results, soak them thoroughly and change the water at least once while cooking them.

532 FIBRE PROVIDERS

For a healthy digestive system, we should aim for an intake of around 20–35g (1–1½oz) of fibre a day, which is equivalent to a couple of pieces of wholemeal bread or a bowl of muesli. Other good dietary sources are vegetables and oats.

533 HUNT OUT HIDDEN CAUSES

One of the major hidden causes of nausea is depression, especially if the nausea and sickness inexplicably last longer than a few days. Make sure that you're giving yourself enough downtime and employ relaxation techniques to ease tension.

534 DON'T DO FAST FOOD

Meals that are eaten in front of the television, at your desk or on the move are more likely to cause nausea and sickness. As an alternative, give yourself some quiet time in a comfortable seat to enjoy chewing and tasting every morsel of your slow food.

535 PRESS YOUR ANTISICKNESS BUTTON

The acupressure point P6 is thought to relieve nausea and travel sickness. It is located between the tendons on the inside arm, three finger widths above the wrist crease. Press lightly for 30 seconds whenever you need relief.

neck stiffness

536 TAKE A SIDEWAYS APPROACH

Inhale and then, as you exhale, slowly lower your right ear towards your right shoulder (it won't reach so don't force it) until there is a gentle stretch along the top of the left shoulder and neck. Take several slow deep breaths. Inhale and raise your head back up. Repeat on the other side.

537 FLEX YOUR NECK

For neck pain and stiffness that have been caused by muscle tightening, gently move the neck to the outer ranges of its movement while sitting in a comfortable chair. This will help release muscle spasms and reduce the associated pain.

538 STRETCH AWAY STIFFNESS

For stiffness, inhale and then, as you exhale, slowly start to lower your chin to your chest, giving yourself a long, gentle stretch along the back of the neck. Take several slow, deep breaths with the chin down and then lift your head back up again on an inhale.

539 ROLL AWAY RIGIDITY

Lower one ear towards your shoulder, then roll your chin down towards the chest, across the chest and up the other side. Inhale and then, as you exhale, roll your chin down across the chest and up the other side.

540 MASSAGE PROBLEMS AWAY

Applying warmth and gentle massage to sore and stiff necks can help reduce pain and increase healing blood flow.

541 SHRUG OFF NECK PROBLEMS

Inhale and raise your shoulders up to your ears, pulling them up as high as they'll go. Then let go with an 'ahhh' and drop your shoulders slowly back down. Repeat several times to ease muscle tension.

542 STAY IN THE SWIM

The best exercise to ease a stiff neck is swimming on your back. The water supports the head without straining the neck, allowing muscles to be used and stretched without discomfort.

543 FORM A SHOULDER CIRCLE

Raise your shoulders up, rotate them back and down, then forwards and up again. Repeat several times, then go in the opposite direction.

544 BE ALERT FOR SYMPTOMS

If your neck pain is ever accompanied by a fever, nausea, swelling or feelings of being generally unwell, you should consult your doctor immediately – the neck pain could be a signpost for several different medical conditions.

pain

545 GIVE YOURSELF A FRUITY FLUSH

Many forms of chronic pain are made worse by indigestion and constipation.
A diet rich in fruit and vegetables loosens stools and prevents pain.

546 LAUGH IT OFF

Laughing – even when you feel like crying from agony – can relax muscles, relieve pain and even boost your immune system. So, the next time you feel a twinge, get the giggles.

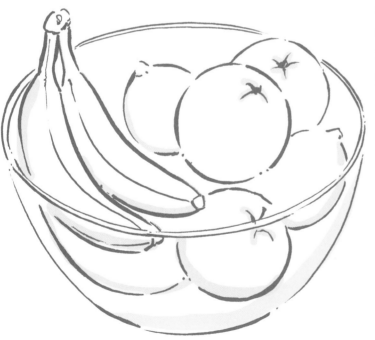

547 RING THE EARACHE CHANGES

The pain of tinnitus – which is often characterized by a constant ringing sound in the ears – can be reduced by taking vitamin B6, found in fruit, vegetables and many supplements.

548 SAY BYE-BYE TO RSI

An estimated one in 50 people suffer some form of RSI (Repetitive Strain Injury), which is caused by repetitive overuse of the soft tissue muscles of the neck, back, shoulders, arms and hands. Most of these injuries could be avoided altogether simply by taking short, regular breaks throughout the day.

549 GET ACTIVE TO GET PAIN-FREE

The last thing you might feel like doing if you're suffering pain is exercise, but gentle activity can actually reduce pain by boosting seratonin levels in the body, which increases the flexibility of blood vessels and reduces pain perception in the brain.

550 BLINK AWAY PAIN

Don't become so transfixed on the screen that you forget to blink. Blinking while watching television or looking at a computer screen will stop your eyes from becoming dry and reduce eye problems and pain as a result.

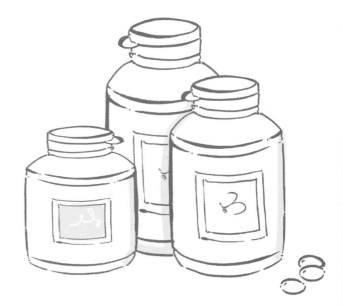

551 THINK YOURSELF SOFT

Focus on the part of your body that is feeling tense or is generating pain. What image comes to mind? Perhaps you see a rock or a tight knot. This represents receptive imagery. Try turning it into something soft, such as clay, or change the colour you perceive it to be, and feel your pain begin to dissolve away.

552 REACH OUT FOR HEALING HANDS

Massage decreases stress hormones, which can be a contributing factor to pain. It also seems to increase levels of endorphins, which are natural painkillers.

553 GO ALL-NATURAL

MSM (methyl-sulphonyl-methane) is an organic form of sulphur that has been shown to alleviate pain without producing side effects. It is found naturally in fruits, vegetables, meat, milk and seafood and seems to be particularly effective at easing muscle cramps.

554 DON'T SKIP MEALS IF YOU WANT TO SKIP PAIN

Skipping meals can result in increased pain, possibly because of fluctuations in blood sugar levels in the body brought on by long periods without nourishment. Always take a healthy snack along with you if you know you will be too busy to make time for a proper meal.

555 MAGNIFY MAGNESIUM

Soya beans, wholegrains, nuts, seeds, vegetables and fish all contain magnesium, which is an effective muscle relaxant shown to reduce tension pain. Lack of magnesium has been linked to depression, muscle soreness and general pain.

556 BLOW HOT AND COLD

Warmth can relieve pain by relaxing muscles. In contrast, cold relieves pain by reducing inflammation. Alternating between the two can help many types of muscle pain.

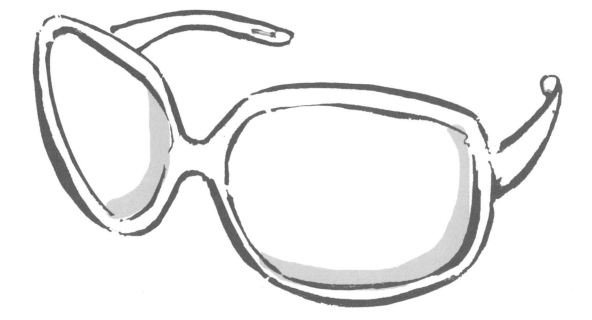

557 INVEST IN SOME SERIOUS SHADES

To prevent eye pain and potential damage, don't skimp on proper eye protection – get a good pair of optical-grade, polarized sunglasses that don't have the distortion associated with some types of cheap lenses. Polarization is essential for cutting glare and reducing eyestrain.

558 PEPPER YOURSELF WITH A CURE

Cayenne pepper contains a substance called capsaicin, which stimulates the brain to secrete endorphins, peptides that help block pain signals and reduce chronic pain, such as that from arthritis and bad backs. Sprinkle the cayenne pepper in hot water for a cure with a kick.

559 SOOTHE SKIN WITH CALENDULA

Calendula is an excellent herb for reducing the pain of most skin disorders, including nappy (diaper) rash, sunburns, bruises, and insect stings and bites. The herb has a calming, soothing effect on irritated skin by reducing inflammation and combating any associated infection, and there are topical skin ointments and creams available.

560 CHECK THE DATE

If soreness and pain are worse at certain times of the month, what you're feeling could be down to your menstrual cycle. Hormonal changes mean that many women are more susceptible to pain in the week before their period commences.

561 BE A PAIN-FREE WATER BABY

Even mild dehydration can trigger pain, so drinking lots of fluids is essential for pain-free living. The head is especially affected, but muscle pain, cramps and eyestrain can be caused by dehydration, too.

562 CATCH UP ON YOUR ZZZZZS

Here is one of the easiest tips for you to try – a good night's sleep is essential for a pain-free life. This is because sleep deprivation causes an increased perception pain. So aim for at least seven hours a night to stay free of pain.

563 FIGHT INFLAMMATION WITH FOOD

Some types of food have natural anti-inflammatory properties that can reduce swelling and, therefore, alleviate pain. The best options for you to try are avocado, banana, berries, cabbage, cucumber, fig, mango and melon.

564 STEER CLEAR OF TRIGGERS

Some types of foods may actually increase the perception of pain, possibly because of their capacity for raising acid levels in the body. So, if you are suffering from persistent pain, cut down on alcohol, coffee, citrus fruits, onions, chocolate, sugar and salt.

stomach problems

565 GO FOR A WALK

Exercise helps move gas through the digestive tract. That's why experts suggest that you take a short walk after eating instead of taking a nap. Mint tea can also aid digestion.

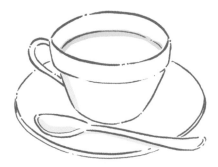

566 SETTLE THE STOMACH WITH MILK

Artichokes and milk products can help indigestion caused by too much stomach acid by lining the inside of the stomach after overeating or excessively rich food.

567 SWAP THE FRIES

French fries, red meat, sugar and refined grains in foods can increase the risk of colon cancer in women who eat them regularly. Replacing these foods with healthier alternatives like wholegrains, boiled or baked potatoes and low-sugar options could help cut your risk of colon cancer by half.

568 GO FOR PEPPER INSTEAD OF MILK TO CURE ULCER PAIN

Calcium in milk could make ulcer pain worse instead of better. To cure ulcers, steer clear of alcohol and spicy foods except capsaicin, a pepper derivative that seems to help ulcer pain.

569 RUB AWAY THE BLOAT

Try stroking gently from your right hip up towards your ribs, across the bottom of your ribcage and down towards your left hip. Repeat several times to encourage the movement of trapped wind.

tired all the time

570 KEEP ZIPPING ALONG

Fatigue is one of the first symptoms of dehydration. Increase your daily intake of water by drinking a glass with each meal and sipping throughout the day.

571 TRASH THE CRASH DIET

Low-calorie consumption is a major cause of fatigue in women today. Those who diet frequently may not have enough fuel to sustain their body's optimal efficiency level, leading to tiredness and fatigue.

572 DON'T COUNT ON CAFFEINE

Caffeine mimics the effects of stress hormones in the body. A person who weighs 70kg (11st/154lb) and drinks more than six caffeine drinks per day (for example, six cups of coffee or cola) can develop caffeine 'poisoning', with symptoms of restlessness, irritability, headache, insomnia and tiredness.

573 CAN TIREDNESS WITH SARDINES

Tiredness can be a result of low iron, which also leads to cracked lips, cold hands and feet, poor memory, headaches, poor resistance to infection and pallor in the face and inner eyelids. Eat iron-rich sardines to boost energy.

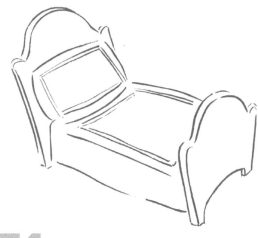

574 DO A SLEEP SURVEY

Lack of sleep or bad-quality sleep is a prime cause of tiredness. Keep track of the hours you sleep and note irregularities. Make sure your room is dark and quiet and don't carry stresses to bed with you.

575 DON'T DISMISS DEPRESSION

One of the major symptoms of depression is extreme tiredness, so if you feel fatigued all the time you might want to consider depression as an underlying cause. Consult your doctor if you need advice.

576 B WISE TO ENERGIZE

Adequate supplies of vitamins and minerals are essential for healthy metabolism. If these become in short supply for any reason, you will soon experience persistent tiredness. The B group of vitamins is especially important, as it's needed to produce energy.

577 ASK THE EXPERTS

If you feel tired all the time (known as TATT) for longer than two weeks, despite increasing exercise levels, eating a healthy diet and improving your quality of sleep, you must see your doctor. Tiredness is an early symptom of many illnesses, including thyroid problems and multiple sclerosis.

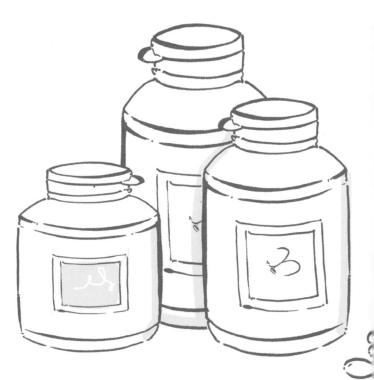

578 DON'T LET HORMONES WEAR YOU OUT

Low oestrogen levels can cause tiredness, especially when hormone levels drop in the week before your period or during the menopause, when tiredness can be overwhelming. Some studies have shown that regular carbohydrate snacks can help prevent this feeling.

579 STUB OUT THE CIGGY

Smoking affects everything to do with your body, increasing dehydration and stress levels and generating a whole range of metabolic problems. Heavy smokers often feel tired due to a lack of oxygen in their bloodstream.

580 LEAP INTO ACTION

Lack of exercise is one of the key causes of low energy and feelings of constant tiredness. Inactivity can also encourage weight gain and this in turn is likely to make you feel depressed.

581 MAKE A MENTAL NOTE

If you are worrying that you haven't completed some chore or important task, make a mental note that you are going to do it and when, which will help your brain stop worrying about it.

582 GET YOUR TIMING RIGHT

Organizing your life better can help you build in more opportunities for relaxation. Aim to balance all the aspects of your life, scheduling in time for your domestic chores and job as well as your social activities.

waterworks

583 DON'T PEE TOO OFTEN

Going to the toilet too frequently can weaken your bladder by causing muscle fatigue, while women who crouch over the toilet are less likely to empty their bladders fully and are at risk of infection.

584 GET IT DOWN TO A TEA

Drinking tea made from raspberry leaves has been shown to reduce the pain and duration of urinary tract infections, and it is especially effective if taken regularly as problems begin.

585 DON'T FORCE IT

If you feel the need to go to the toilet but once you get there you're as dry as a bone, you could have a urinary tract infection. Consult your doctor straight away in order to prevent the problem spreading to the bladder and kidneys and becoming even more serious.

586 JACK IN THE PACK

Smoking increases the risk of urinary tract conditions as well as raises blood pressure and stimulates coughing, which can add to problems with bladder control. It also increases the risk of bladder cancer, a risk that can stay with you for years after you have quit smoking.

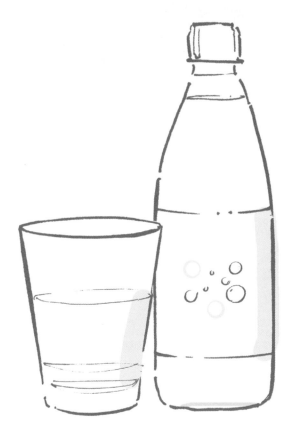

587 GET THE ALL-CLEAR

Aim to drink enough water to make your urine pale yellow and clear. Dark yellow or cloudy urine is a sign that you aren't consuming enough fluid, so drink up.

588 STAY OFF STRONG STIMULANTS

Coffee, alcohol, spicy foods, citrus fruits and chocolate can all aggravate bladder problems, making urine more concentrated and so forcing the body to expend water in order to detoxify itself.

589 SIT DOWN AFTER SEX

During sexual intercourse, bacteria may enter the urethra. By going to the toilet straight afterwards, you help wash out the invaders right away and avoid infections.

590 WIPE AWAY PROBLEMS

Keep infections at bay by cleaning the vaginal area with a front-to-back motion, which helps prevent the spread of bacteria from the anus.

591 HALT THE FLOW TO STAY STRONG BELOW

When you pee, practise stopping and starting the flow using your pelvic floor muscles to keep them tight and strong, Don't overdo it, though – three times a day is enough to help build muscle strength.

592 AVOID THE FIZZ

Fizzy mineral water can exacerbate some urinary tract conditions, so if you want to stay pain-free, have plenty of still, clear water to flush out the problems.

593 CHOOSE CRANBERRIES FOR CYSTITIS

Women have known this for years, but drinking cranberry juice regularly can help ease the symptoms of cystitis, possibly because it alters the acidity levels of the urine.

594 EAT TO CURE URINARY INFECTIONS

Health-inducing blueberries are rich in the bacteria-killing anthocyanosides, which will also see off the dreaded *E. coli* infections by preventing the infectious bacteria from clinging to the cells that line the urinary tract and bladder.

menopause

595 EAT YOUR GREENS

Postmenopausal women who have an excess of animal foods in their diet are more likely to have low bone density, because of the high acid levels in meat. Vegetables will counteract the acidity of meaty dishes, so it's important to eat a balanced diet.

596 HERBAL REMEDY FOR HOT FLUSHES

The herbal supplement black cohosh has been found to alleviate menopausal symptoms, such as hot flushes, sleep disturbance and depressive moods, when taken daily.

597 STAY SOYA STRONG

Menopausal women who eat soya benefit from a noticeable lessening of upsetting symptoms as well as a lower risk of bone disease because of the bone-strengthening effects of the food.

588 DON'T SWEAT IT WITH YOGA

Yoga and the Alexander Technique can reduce menopausal symptoms such as hot flushes and night sweats, while relaxation techniques, such as meditation and visualization, may assist by relieving mental and physical stress.

589 COOL DOWN WITH VITAMINS

Many women claim to have experienced beneficial effects from taking vitamin E for hot flushes and vitamin B2 for headaches.

600 MINIMIZE MOOD SWINGS

St John's Wort is effective in treating mood swings as well as mild depression. Liquorice is thought to help hot flushes but it can increase blood pressure so, as with all herbal preparations, use it with caution.

601 SPARE THE SPICE

Avoid foods and drinks that may trigger hot flushes, such as spicy cuisine, citrus fruits, alcohol and caffeine.

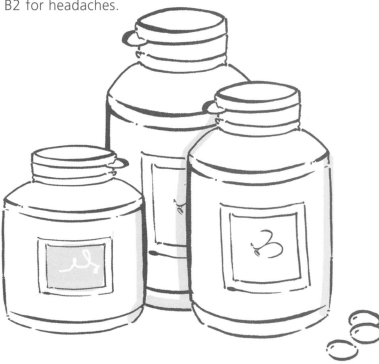

602 POP CORN TO POP DEPRESSION

A slight drop in the levels of the 'feel good' brain chemical serotonin could be one of the causes of depression during the menopause. A high-carbohydrate, low-fat snack, such as fat-free popcorn, may help restore serotonin levels in the brain, thereby improving your mood.

603 NATURAL HRT

Phytoestrogens are oestrogen-like compounds that are found in soya beans. They seem to bind to oestrogen receptors and act in a similar way to the female hormone in the body, reducing the incidence of hot flushes by up to 40%.

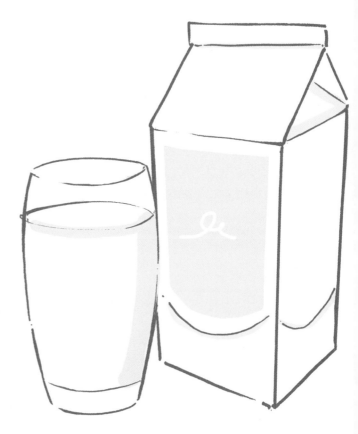

604 BE A COOL SNACKER

Eat small, frequent meals instead of fewer, large meals, which can dilate the blood vessels and increase the probability of hot flushes and skin reddening.

605 HAVE FUN WITH FUNGUS

Mushrooms, as well as onions, milk, garlic, eggs and seafood, contain selenium, which is an antioxidant mineral that can alleviate menopausal distress and allow you to smile through the flushes.

periods

606 JOG AWAY PAIN

Taking regular exercise – for example, aerobics or jogging – can help reduce the symptoms of PMS (PMT). However, you should be exercising on a regular basis, not just when symptoms are present, if you want to enjoy the full health benefits.

607 STAY CHASTE TO CHASE PAIN AWAY

Chasteberry, which is also known as vitex agnus-castus, regulates female hormonal imbalances in the body by working on the pituitary gland in the brain, helping with PMS (PMT) irritability, breast pain and water retention.

608 TAKE YOUR FINGER OFF THE STRESS TRIGGER

Pinpointing and avoiding any emotional triggers or stresses that make the symptoms of PMS (PMT) worse, and discussing these with your partner or a friend and asking for their support, can be useful ways to avoid problems.

609 JUST B HAPPY

Some women have found that taking vitamin B (particularly B6) is helpful in reducing PMS (PMT) symptoms, but there is only limited scientific evidence that this works, and high doses can cause damage to the nervous system.

610 SMOOTHIE AWAY SYMPTOMS

Studies suggest that daily doses of magnesium and calcium taken during the time PMS (PMT) symptoms occur could have a cocktail of effects – helping reduce mood swings, muscle pains and fluid retention. Get both minerals at once in a soothing banana smoothie, made with either milk or yogurt.

611 EXPERIMENT WITH EPO

Some women find that taking evening primrose oil helps relieve breast discomfort. Long-term treatment (more than three months) may be required before any effect is noticed, however.

612 SECURE A FISHY CURE

Fish fats help to relieve the symptoms of premenstrual disorders, including breast pain, PMT, bloating, depression and irritability. Choose oily fish such as mackerel, herring, sardines and salmon for the best effects.

613 IRON OUT PMT PROBLEMS

Heavy menstrual blood flow can deplete your body's iron stores, which can in turn cause further bleeding. Women who increase the iron in their diets are likely to suffer less heavy and painful periods. Sources include lean red meat, sardines, egg yolk, dried figs and dark green leafy vegetables like spinach.

614 YOU CAN BE TOO THIN

When it comes to weight loss, your periods prove it is possible to be too thin. Beware of dieting so much that your menstrual cycle is affected, as too much weight loss can make periods stop and affect fertility.

615 PLANT THE SEEDS OF A CURE

Blackcurrant seeds, evening primrose seeds and borage seeds are all high in gamma linolenic acid (GLA), which helps regulate fluid retention and hormone release, helping minimize symptoms of PMS (PMT) and period problems.

616 SEND PMT CRAMPS BALMY

Lemonbalm is often used for menstrual problems as it has a calming and regulating effect in the menstrual cycle. It helps ease menstrual cramps and treats irregularities.

617 BEEF UP TO REDUCE CRAMPS

Supplementing the diet with zinc, found in high proportions in red meats like beef and lamb, has been found to reduce cramps, bloating and other PMS (PMT) symptoms.

618 STRENGTHEN WITH VITAMIN C

Taking vitamin C and bioflavonoids may strengthen uterine blood vessels and make them less susceptible to damage, so reducing the severity and length of bleeding during periods.

619 MANAGE WITH MARJORAM

Essential oil of marjoram has been shown to increase warmth and comfort if used to massage the abdomen during menstruation or in a burner to encourage pain-free sleep.

620 CURB PAIN WITH A HERB

Eating the common garden herb feverfew can lessen cramping, headaches, neck and shoulder pain and muscle soreness during menstruation by acting as a natural painkiller. Make yourself a sandwich or salad garnished with feverfew or a herbal tea from the leaves.

621 SWAP FATS TO PREVENT WATER RETENTION

Low-fat diets could not only reduce water retention in the week before your period commences but also lessen the severity of the period itself. Fish oils are a great choice because they will also work to reduce PMS (PMT) symptoms.

622 MASSAGE AWAY THE PAIN

Place your hands on your hips with the thumbs on the lower back at hip level, either side of the spine, and move the thumbs in small, light circular motions. Be gentle to avoid pain or discomfort.

623 GIVE THE G-STRING THE BOOT

Swapping your G-string or thong for bigger underwear could help banish such thong-related problems as folliculitis, thrush, redness and soreness. Choose thicker varieties of underwear made in natural, breathable fabrics such as cotton, or go commando during exercise, when they cause most friction problems.

pregnancy

624 DROP THE DRINK

Research has shown that during the early stages of pregnancy, women drinking 10 units of alcohol on a single occasion were more likely to have a child with a congenital abnormality than those who drank more moderately. Alcohol consumption of more than three drinks per week roughly doubles your chance of having a miscarriage.

625 DON'T EAT FOR TWO

Experts recommend that pregnant women need only an extra 300 calories a day to ensure the proper development of the foetus, and then only in the last three months. Energy requirements change little during pregnancy, so the effects of eating those extra calories are likely just to add weight to the mother.

626 SEAFOOD FOR A GOOD BIRTHWEIGHT BABY

Low consumption of seafood during the early stages of pregnancy may be a strong risk factor for low birthweight, because the omega-3 fatty acids they contain may help foetal development.

627 FOCUS ON FOLIC ACID

Folic acid lowers the chances that your baby will have spinal cord problems, so pregnant women should take a daily supplement before and during pregnancy until the twelfth week.

628 SWIM AWAY FROM PAIN

Swimming can help relieve many aches and pains and makes you feel weightless. This reduces pressure on the joints, hips and spine, which can become sore in the later months of pregnancy.

629 DON'T CURB CARBS

Mothers who eat more carbohydrates than fats while they're breast-feeding may have higher levels of a hormone known as leptin in their blood, which may later help them lose any weight that they gained during pregnancy. Carbohydrates are also essential for producing breastmilk.

630 TAKE VITAMINS TO VANQUISH TOXINS

Vitamins C and E fight off the symptoms of pre-eclampsia, a serious pregnancy-related condition that generates toxic compounds, raises blood pressure and endangers the life of mother and child. In studies, women taking a combined supplement had a 76% lower risk of developing the condition.

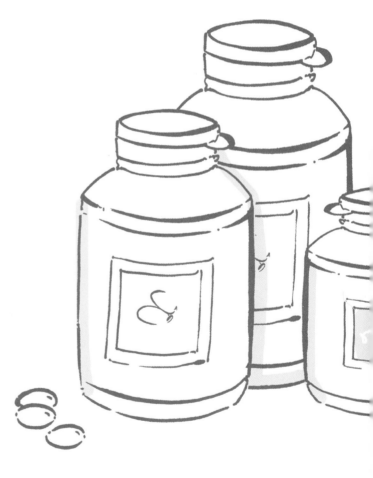

631 CHOCOLATE FOR A HAPPY BABY

Women who eat chocolate during their pregnancy have babies who are happier and healthier than the children of mothers who abstain, possibly thanks to the mood-boosting chemicals it contains.

632 SNIFF AWAY LABOUR PAINS

Anxiety, pain, nausea and vomiting during labour can all be helped by using aromatherapy. The scents of ginger and citrus fruits are good for nausea, while bergamot, eucalyptus and pine are thought to lessen pain.

633 STRETCH OUT TIRED BACKS

The leg lift crawl is excellent for an aching back. To do this, kneel on your hands and knees. Slowly bring your right knee towards your right elbow. Then slowly straighten your leg and lift it up and back, parallel to the floor. Avoid sudden jerks and keep your back straight, not arched. Repeat with each leg five to ten times.

634 SAY CHEESE

Calcium is vital for a healthy pregnancy so make sure you include pasteurized cheese, milk or yogurt in your diet, as well as dark green vegetables.

635 BE A WHITE WITCH

Witch hazel lotion and gel can reduce the pain and swelling of haemorrhoids. For further relief, try warm baths or use witch hazel compresses to ease severe swelling.

636 STARCH AWAY MORNING SICKNESS

Include more starchy foods in your diet, such as rice, potatoes, soda crackers and toast, as these can soothe an upset stomach. Make sure you eat soon after waking to prevent the onset of sickness.

637 KEEP IT MOVING

Gentle exercise will help you stay in shape during pregnancy, can lower your risk of miscarriage and has been proven to help reduce labour complications and length.

638 TILT YOUR PELVIS LIKE ELVIS

Taking exercise in the form of gentle pelvic tilts, using the muscles of your lower abdomen, will help relieve compression pain in your lower back, and it may even encourage the baby to assume a good birth position.

639 BRUSH UP ON TOOTHCARE

Take extra care of your general oral hygiene, especially your teeth and gums, during pregnancy as they may become more prone to plaque, cavities and disease at this time. Daily flossing and regular brushing after meals with a soft-to-medium brush is the answer.

640 CAVE IN TO CRAVINGS

There is some evidence to suggest that food cravings may be your body's way of ensuring you get the vitamins and minerals you lack during pregnancy. So giving in to them might not be a bad thing – as long as you don't overeat.

641 WALK ON SUNSHINE

Taking a brisk walk – which means covering 1.5km (1 mile) in about 12 to 15 minutes – several times a week is an excellent form of exercise before, during and after pregnancy. In addition, walking outdoors in good weather ensures that you will get a healthy dose of daily sunlight, which not only boosts vitamin D levels but also improves your mood.

642 TAKE IT EASY AT THE START

For the first three months, pregnant women should avoid overexertion and dehydration as this is a critical time for the baby and these conditions could harm development or trigger miscarriage.

643 BE A DAIRY LOVER

Regularly drinking more milk, or foods that substitute for milk, and eating more protein will help your baby's development in the womb by keeping your calcium at optimum level.

cellulite

644 DRINK AWAY YOUR DIMPLES

Much cellulite is thought to be the result of an insufficient water intake. Drinking water plumps up the skin cells and smooths out subcutaneous dimpling. So if you want the smoothest possible skin, you should drink eight glasses a day.

645 FIGHT FAT TO FIGHT CELLULITE

Cellulite is simply fat under the skin that has a dimpled appearance. It looks this way because women have a layer of irregular and discontinuous connective tissue immediately below the skin. If you lose fat, you'll lose cellulite, too.

646 DON'T CRASH AND BURN

Crash diets don't banish cellulite – in fact, they increase the risk because the body goes into starvation mode and holds on to fat, particularly in storage areas like the thighs and hips.

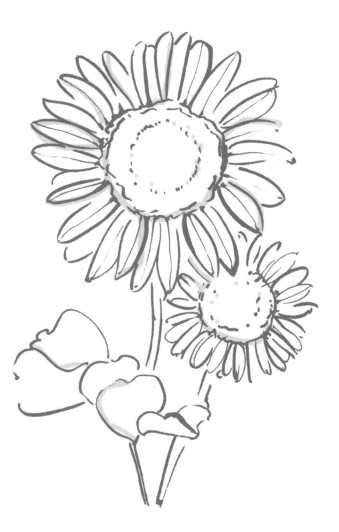

647 USE SUNFLOWERS TO SHRINK FAT

Fluid retention can result in the development of cellulite, as fluids become trapped in the fatty cells located under the skin. Linoleic acid, which is a substance found in sunflower and corn oils, may lessen fluid retention and so improve the appearance of cellulite.

648 RELAX FOR REALLY GOOD SKIN

Tension and stress can cause a muscle to seize up and contract and they can do the same for connective tissues (the same effect as if you squeeze a fatty area), increasing the uneven effect of fat under the skin.

649 GIVE TOXINS THE BRUSH OFF

Body brushing until the skin turns pink improves circulation to fatty areas, where blood flow is less efficient than in other areas of the body. This helps provide energy for healing and boosts the waste-removal process.

650 QUIT THE WEED TO SMOKE OUT DIMPLES

Smoking weakens the skin by causing constriction of the blood capillaries, worsening circulation and damaging the connective tissues, which in turn causes the dimpling effect of cellulite. Quit smoking to quash cellulite.

651 KEEP YOURSELF STIMULATED

Rubbing coffee grounds on areas affected by cellulite might be the supermodel's favourite trick, but it doesn't have to be coffee. The benefits are due to the skin stimulation, which boosts circulation and works toxins away from fatty areas.

652 GO GREEN TO BURN AWAY FAT

Studies have shown that drinking three cups of green tea a day can help reduce cellulite by boosting baseline metabolism and helping the body eliminate toxins. The caffeine it contains has a further stimulating effect.

653 WORK IT OUT

Exercise not only promotes overall health, but also works to improve muscle tone and circulation and frees up blocked tissue to remove the appearance of cellulite.

654 PILL A FAST ONE

Contraceptive pills raise oestrogen levels and can make fat cells enlarge and retain water, leading to cellulite. Diuretics, diet and sleeping pills can all make it worse.

655 GIVE CAFFEINE THE THUMBS UP

Some have claimed that caffeine and spicy foods add toxins to the body, which causes cellulite formation, but there is no evidence for this. In fact, caffeine might help get rid of cellulite by stimulating fat burning.

656 GO LEAN FOR THINNER THIGHS

Saturated fats build cellulite and block arteries, and they can get trapped in the body's tissues, preventing waste and toxin elimination and encouraging fatty deposits.

657 GIVE YOURSELF A HELPING HAND

Massaging your thighs and hips can help promote circulation to fatty areas. Make sure the massage strokes always travel upwards, towards the heart – in the direction of lymph clearance.

658 DON'T RELY ON DIET ALONE

People who exercise as well as diet to get thinner lose more subcutaneous fat (the fat that appears as cellulite) than people who only diet. Studies show that the more often you work out, the slimmer you'll get.

hair & scalp

659 DRY BRUSH BEFORE BEDTIME

For the healthiest hair, avoid brushing when hair is wet, sticking instead to a wide-toothed comb to ease out knots. Instead, dry brush the whole head at night to stimulate growth and oil production.

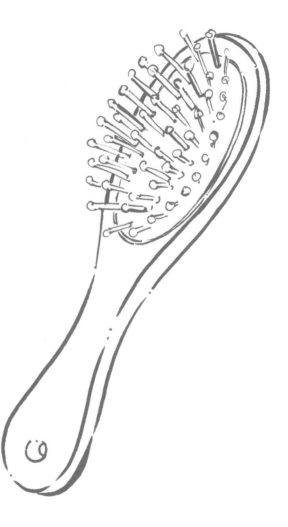

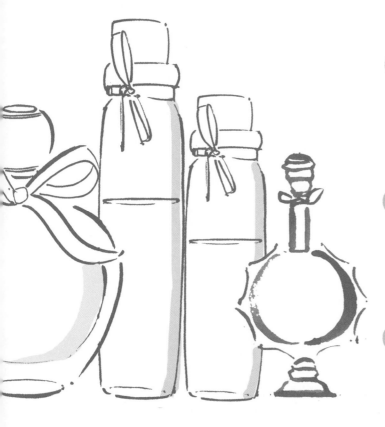

660 DITCH THE ITCH

Ease an itchy, flaky scalp with a relaxing tea tree oil head massage to stimulate circulation in the scalp and help clear up dry and itchy skin.

661 RINSE, RINSE AND RINSE AGAIN

Many people confuse dried hair product with dandruff. For a healthy scalp, avoid heavy styling products and rinse thoroughly to avoid buildup.

662 STOP FLAKEOUTS WITH FOOD

To avoid the flake, steer clear of too much spicy food, alcohol and dairy products. Experts say stress is also a big cause of dandruff, especially around the hairline.

663 FIGHT THE FRIZZ

Coconut oil reduces frizziness and dryness in lacklustre hair, not only when used as a hair treatment but also when eaten. Coconut can be flaked or shredded and coconut milk can be used in cooking.

664 FISH FOR SHINIER HAIR

Eating fish regularly helps your hair by strengthening roots and boosting shine by encouraging natural oil production.

665 SHINE UP WITH SWEET POTATO

Sweet potato, carrot and red pepper contain high levels of betacarotene, which the body needs to create vitamin A, essential to provide a protective layer to the outside of hair strands.

666 GET AHEAD WITH SOYA

Soya not only boosts hair health but has also been shown to make hair grow faster at the root and strengthen the shaft against damage.

667 MASSAGE FOR THICKER HAIR

Thinning hair and a lazy scalp can be stimulated by a weekly scalp massage. Use fingertips to rub small areas of the scalp at a time, remembering to include the hair-line, where dead skin cells can build up.

hands & feet

668 GO FLAT OUT

Researchers have found that constant wearing of high-heeled shoes can cause joint problems in the long term because weight is thrown onto the ball of the foot. Choose lower heels or trainers for a healthier walk, or alternate stilettos with kitten heels if you can't give them up.

669 BLISTERING HEALTH

Studies have shown that piercing a blister in the first three hours can help it heal. Use a sterile needle and lance as shallowly as possible in two places from opposite sides, treating to avoid infection.

670 ROLL AWAY STRESSFUL FEET

Feet can take a pounding during the day and a great way to relieve stress when you get home from work is to roll your feet over a cold soft-drink can to stimulate blood flow and reduce swelling.

671 LOOK AT YOUR FEET FOR INSULIN BALANCE

The condition and appearance of your feet can be a valuable indicator of more general health problems, including diabetes. If, for example, your feet look swollen and red, or they are infected, painful, tingling or numb, you should seek medical advice.

672 SOFTEN OFTEN

The secret of dealing with hard skin on feet is to rub it away every day rather than at the odd irregular session. Use a pumice stone or file, softening the skin first by soaking in water with a teaspoon of bicarbonate of soda.

673 REACH FOR SOME LEMON AID

The citric acid in lemon juice works as a natural bleaching agent for discoloured nail tips. Dip a cotton bud (swab) in neat lemon juice and work it under the nail, then rinse after ten minutes for super-clean nails.

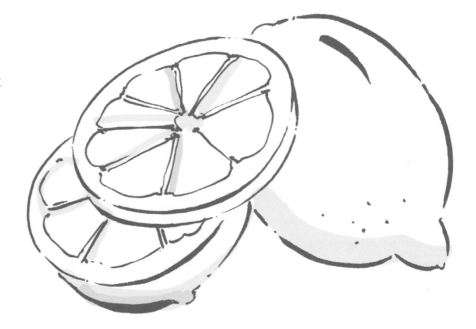

674 GO FORMALDEHYDE-FREE

If you have brittle nails, don't use polish or treatments with formaldehyde. Instead soak your nails for ten minutes in wheatgerm or olive oil, massaging it into the cuticles.

675 FOIL FLAKINESS WITH STARFLOWER OIL

Flaky nails can be sprung back into health by including starflower or evening primrose oil in the diet or as a supplement. Both contain the essential fatty acids (EFAs) necessary for the structure of cells.

676 IRON OUT FLAT NAILS

Too little iron in the diet can lead to thin, flat nails so increase your iron intake by eating foods such as lean red meat, dried fruit and nuts and green vegetables.

677 CHECK YOUR RIDGES

Ridges running across your nails could be a sign that stress is affecting your body in adverse ways. If your nails feel rippled, think about giving yourself time to relax.

678 BRUSH UP FOR CLEAN HANDS

Brushing your fingertips with toothpaste can remove nicotine or ink stains. Use a nailbrush to work the toothpaste into the skin for a few minutes, then rinse off.

679 ALLOW NAILS TO BREATHE

A couple of days a month give your nails some time off polish so they can breathe. Buffing during this time will give them a natural shine and boost circulation.

680 USE FINGERTIP MASSAGE

Massaging a nail and cuticle cream or oil into your nails every night helps the fingertips retain moisture. If you use one infused with lavender, it could help you fall asleep, too.

681 GET PRIMROSE-STRONG NAILS

Evening primrose oil is essential for strong, hardy nails, and getting enough calcium, iron, zinc, protein and vitamins A, B and C is important as well.

682 CLOCK THOSE SOCKS!

Feet perspire more than any other area of the body, with each foot containing around 25,000 sweat glands and producing an eggcup of sweat every day. Wearing socks in natural or wicking materials helps them stay dry and healthy.

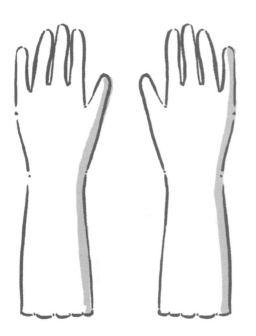

683 WATCH OUT FOR CLUBBING

Clubbing is when fingertips widen and become round, with nails curved around the fingertips. This serious condition is the result of an enlargement in connective tissue and can be a sign of an underlying lung disease. You must consult your doctor for advice.

684 DON'T FILE AWAY STRENGTH

Avoid filing your nails as much as you possibly can, and, when you have to file, always do it in one direction only. To help your nails, wear gloves when washing dishes and doing other household chores and keep exposure to harsh chemicals, especially bleach, to a minimum.

685 STOP NAIL BREAKS

Everyone's nails grow about 3mm (⅛in) per month. However, most people do not see anything like that growth, not because their nails are slow but because they tend to break off regularly.

686 WATCH OUT FOR BEAU'S LINES

Beau's lines are indentations that run across the nail and appear when growth at the matrix is disturbed. This can happen after illness or prolonged periods of stress.

687 GO FISHY TO CURE WHITE SPOTS

Eat foods rich in sulphur and silicon, such as broccoli, fish, royal jelly, kelp and onions, which will help preserve nail colour and keep cuticles pink and strong.

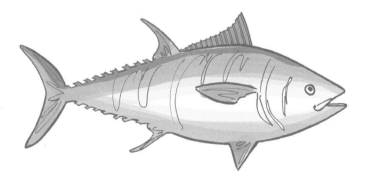

688 PUSH THE RIGHT BUTTONS

Nails and fingertips can suffer when in constant contact with keyboards for typing. Give them a rest by stretching out hands and shaking fingers to reduce tension.

689 KEEP IT TOGETHER

When the nail separates from the nail bed, this can be a sign that something is wrong, such as psoriasis, fungal infection, contact dermatitis or an adverse drug reaction. It can also be a sign of thyroid problems.

690 BITE BACK THE BITING

Don't be tempted to bite and chew your nails. Not only does this cause splits and tears in otherwise healthy nails, it can also transmit infection from mouth bacteria and open up tiny tears in the nail bed. Try chewing gum instead.

681 AVOID THE CUT

Never cut cuticles, because they will only grow back thicker if you snip them off. Instead, warm up hands in warm water or steam and gently push back cuticles with a cuticle stick.

682 DON'T DIG UP TROUBLE

Don't dig under nails to clean them, which damages the thin protective underlayer. Instead, use a soft nailbrush or an old toothbrush to get to hard-to-reach areas.

skin health

683 EAT FISH TO FIGHT FLAKY SKIN

Flaky, dry skin could signal that you are not getting enough essential fatty acids (EFAs), found in certain fish, seeds, nuts and oils. Healthy skin should contain about 15% fatty acids, so make sure you eat at least four portions of EFA-rich foods a week.

694 C IS FOR COLLAGEN

Vitamin C is essential for the growth of new collagen, which keeps the structure of your skin supple and firm and young-looking. Without it, skin will start to sag and look tired and old. So make sure you get enough in your diet and stop smoking, as it reduces vitamin C absorption.

695 DECREASE STRESS TO DEGREASE

Greasy skin can be triggered by hormone changes during times of stress, when the adrenal gland is stimulated into producing more sebum. Cutting out fried food and saturated fats from your diet in favour of fruit and vegetables can help, as can relaxation and destressing.

696 QUIT SMOKING TO KEEP SKIN SUPPLE

Smokers have saggier skin than non-smokers because of the damage done to their skin's elastin by the oxidative elements found in smoke, and because smoking impedes circulation.

697 ANTIOXIDANTS TO FIGHT AGEING

Antioxidants in vitamin A (sources include vegetables and fruit such as tomatoes, carrots, sweet potatoes, watermelons and apricots) combat free radicals that may lead to premature skin ageing and disease.

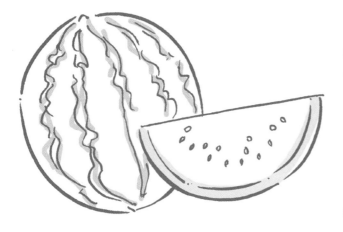

698 ZAP STRESS TO CURE ZITS

Pimples, especially if located around the temples and forehead, could indicate stress. Make sure you drink lots of water and try to relax more.

699 SEED THE DIFFERENCE

The omega-6 fats, which are derived exclusively from seeds and their oils, are essential for skin health, keeping it firm and moisturized. The best sources of omega-6 fats are hemp, pumpkin, sunflower, sesame, walnut and primrose oils, which can be included in the diet or as an element in beauty regimes.

700 KEEP IT CLEAN

Spots and pimples around the chin or jaw may well be due to hormones, and might occur as part of your menstrual cycle. Make sure your skin is kept clean and they should soon disappear.

701 TREAT PALE SKIN WITH IRON

Nearly 18% of women suffer from a lack of iron. If the skin appears pale and thin, this could be the problem. The richest sources are red meat, tuna and sardines, and the body also has the ability to convert lentils into iron.

702 ATTACK ACNE WITH PRIMROSE OIL

Take linseed (flaxseed) oil or evening primrose oil – which are both good sources of essential fatty acids (EFAs) – every day to rebalance the skin oils and to prevent the excess sebum production that can result in the development of acne.

703 WITCH HUNT FOR HEALTHY SKIN

Witch hazel has anti-inflammatory properties that can help soothe and heal minor skin irritations, inflammation of the skin and mucous membranes, varicose veins and haemorrhoids when applied directly, and gum problems when diluted as a mouth rinse.

704 E-LIMINATE DERMATITIS

Atopic dermatitis, a skin disorder characterized by redness, itching, eczema and thickening of the skin, can be soothed and even cured by a daily dose of the antioxidant vitamin E, found in avocado, seeds, nuts and supplements.

705 EAT AWAY SPOTS AND INFECTIONS

Zinc is essential for a healthy immune system and for fighting spots and skin blemishes. Found in red meat, oysters, peanuts and sunflower seeds, this mineral helps reduce the risk of skin infections, spots and boils.

706 SCRATCH THE BOOZE TO CURE THE ITCH

Psoriasis, a skin condition where the skin develops itchy red spots and patches, has been shown to be exacerbated by alcohol, perhaps owing to its dehydrating effects. If you drink, make sure you keep your water levels up.

707 TRY TEA TREE

Tea tree oil can help relieve acne and is also active against other skin problems, including fungal infections and cuts, bruises and bites. Manuka honey – made from tea tree sap – is also a powerful antiseptic with moisturizing qualities.

708 B GOOD TO YOUR SKIN

Vitamin B3 is an essential vitamin for healthy skin. Found in wholemeal bread and other wholegrain products, enriched breads and cereals, beef, chicken, nuts, peanut butter and salmon, it will help skin stay supple.

709 PINCH FOR YOUNG SKIN

The skin-elasticity test is a good measure of how young your skin looks. Pinch the skin on the back of your hand for five seconds then count how long it takes to flatten back out. Average age rates are ten seconds for a 60-year-old, five seconds for a 50-year-old and one second for a 20-year-old.

710 GO BLACK TO BASICS

Blackcurrant oil contains high levels of gamma linolenic acid (GLA), which promotes healthy, fast growth of skin, hair and nails. Use daily but expect to wait up to six weeks before you see visible results.

711 GET CITRUS-SMOOTH SKIN

Lemons and limes are good sources of vitamin C, which protects the skin against ageing. The pith is rich in bioflavonoids, which help strengthen the tiny blood capillaries in the skin and prevent those unattractive broken veins.

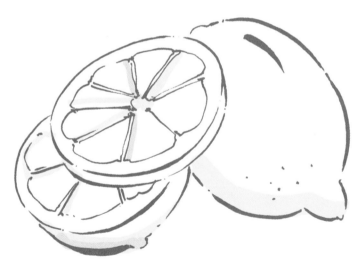

712 BE ROUGH TO BE SMOOTH

Exfoliation boosts blood flow to the skin, helps the skin renewal process and gets rid of dry skin cells that block and dull the complexion. Exfoliate with a gentle granular scrub once a week for the best results.

713 VOTE GREEN

Green tea, whether drunk or used as an ointment, reduces inflammatory responses and can help prevent skin problems.

714 GET A ROSY GLOW

Rosa mosqueta oil reduces scarring and blemishes, and can also help smooth wrinkles and plump up the skin's moisture levels to give it a natural, rosy glow.

715 AVOID THE SQUEEZE

Squeezing spots might be tempting, but it can push the acne plug deeper into the skin and damage the follicle, leading to scars. Instead, apply tea tree oil or aloe vera to soothe.

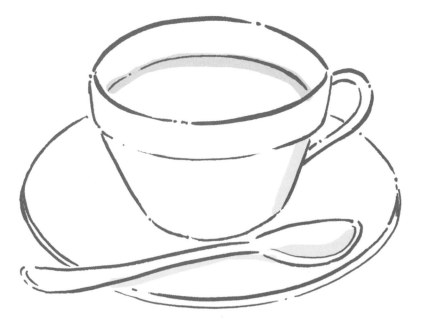

716 GET A-GRADE SKIN

Foods that contain high levels of vitamin A, such as sweet potatoes, carrots, melons, red peppers, spinach, tomatoes, liver, fish, egg yolks, milk and other dairy products, boost general skin health and encourage regeneration of new skin.

717 LIQUIDIZE TO LICK SKIN INFECTION

Try this tip. Juice 4 carrots, 2 asparagus spears, half an iceberg lettuce and a handful of spinach leaves to protect your skin against infections and to maintain its suppleness. Drink this concoction three times a week.

718 REPLICATE HIGH-TECH RETINOL

Retinol, which is the magic ingredient of expensive antiageing creams, is a form of vitamin A. Get your dose from the retinol in animal foods such as liver, oily fish, egg yolk, butter and cheese. The body converts retinol to vitamin A to build up collagen in deep skin layers.

719 DIAGNOSE DRY SKIN

A condition like extremely dry skin could be an indicator of an underlying health problem such as diabetes, which causes circulation problems and can cause the skin to flake and dry. If you are worried, seek medical advice.

720 NOURISH SKIN WITH NUTS

Both walnuts and almonds are high in essential fatty acids (EFAs), which help replenish collagen, naturally moisturize the skin and promote youthful skin firmness. These nuts also contain anti-inflammatory properties that help keep skin smooth and pimple-free.

721 SWEAT OUT IMPURITIES

Adequate water intake not only means the skin can boost moisture naturally, it also allows for constant perspiration through tiny sweat glands. Dehydration can stop this flow of water through the body and lead to spots and pimples.

722 BE A VIRGIN BEAUTY QUEEN

Extra-virgin olive oil contains strong antioxidants that combat the oxidizing effects of the sun on skin, reducing the signs of damage and ageing. Applying olive oil to the skin after sun exposure may help protect it.

723 EXERCISE YOUR SKIN INTO SHAPE

Exercise promotes blood flow, taking nutrients to the skin's surface. Thanks to blood being pumped around the body, live skin cells lying deep in the skin are pushed up higher to the surface, ensuring a healthy renewal process.

724 GET YOUR BEAUTY SLEEP

Beauty sleep is not a myth. While you sleep, your skin regenerates and repairs itself. The peak time for moisture loss is 11pm to 4am. Older skin especially can suffer cell death if too much moisture evaporates, so make sure you go to bed well moisturized so the skin can heal itself.

725 SHIELD SKIN WITH SHEA

Shea butter contains incredibly high levels of vitamin E, which prevents oxidative damage to skin when applied regularly.

726 DON'T YO-YO

Drastic weight fluctuations can stretch out the skin and cause it to sag. Avoid putting on or dropping too much weight for the best-looking skin long-term.

727 LOOK AFTER THIN SKIN

The skin on your face is the thinnest on the body, and the older the skin, the thinner and drier it can be. It will therefore need more protection and moisture, especially in the harsh winter months.

728 OXYGENATE WITH GREEN LEAFYS

Like other green leafy vegetables, kale is rich in the antioxidant lutein and contains iron, which transports oxygen to your skin. It also contains vitamin A, which helps prevent premature wrinkling.

728 HEAL YOUR SKIN WITH PEPPERS

Both red and dark orange peppers are loaded with the antioxidant vitamins A and E and bioflavonoids, which help skin to heal from within.

730 OIL UP WRINKLES WITH SALMON

Along with other coldwater fish like mackerel and tuna, salmon are rich in omega-3 fatty acids, which prevent inflammation and lubricate your skin.

sun safety

731 BEWARE OF AROMATHERAPY OILS

Some types of oils, including citrus oils like orange, lemon and bergamot, react with ultraviolet light from the sun and can cause skin to burn more easily, so beware of using them during summer months.

732 VITAL VITAMIN PROTECTION

Vitamins C and E may help protect the skin against sunburn and could possibly reduce the risk of skin cancer by neutralizing damaging free radicals that are produced by ultraviolet radiation coming from sunlight.

733 KEEP KIDS UNDER COVER

Most people receive up to 80% of their total lifetime exposure to the sun during their first 18 years of life, when skin is most susceptible to sun damage. Just one severe case of sunburn during childhood can double the risk of developing skin cancer later in life.

734 BE A COVER GIRL

Covering up your skin with clothing, wearing sunglasses and wide-brimmed hats to protect the eyes and face, and using sunscreen with an SPF of 15 or more can help prevent damage from the sun and protect against skin cancer.

735 DON'T GO OUT IN THE MIDDAY SUN

Staying inside during the sun's peak hours, between 11am and 2pm, or taking cover under shade from trees or umbrellas during this time, can help prevent skin damage because this is when the sun's UVA rays are at their strongest.

736 TOP IT UP FOR TIP-TOP PROTECTION

Waterproof sunscreens, which cannot be washed off by water or removed as you sweat, should be applied about 30 minutes before exposure to the sun and then reapplied every two hours while you're exposed to direct sunlight.

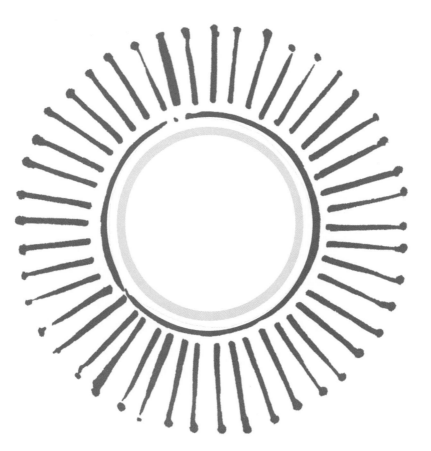

737 OPT FOR TOTAL COVER

When you're applying sunscreen, always remember not to miss hands, neck, ears and lips, which are common sites for skin cancer because of their propensity to burn.

728 KEEP YOUNG AND BEAUTIFUL

After smoking, sun exposure is the greatest wrinkle-creator for skin. Stay out of the sun or use moisturizing sunscreens with a high SPF factor to maximize your skin's chances of staying healthy and youthful.

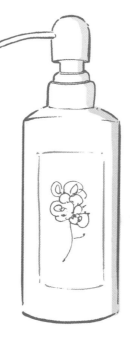

teeth

738 BE A SOFT TOUCH

Lots of gum problems are caused by brushing too vigorously, which can cause gums to retreat. Electric toothbrushes can tackle this by preventing hard pressing. If you're using a normal toothbrush, remember that bristles should bend only slightly against the tooth surface.

740 FLOSS AWAY DECAY

If you don't floss, you will leave an incredible 35% of the surface of your teeth completely untouched and uncleaned. So for really clean teeth, use thick tape and floss every night.

741 GUM IT UP

Chewing sugarfree gum increases saliva flow, which helps neutralize plaque acidity and helps teeth stay healthy. But too much gum-chewing can cause gas, so stick to one pack a day at most.

742 KEEP CLEAR OF BAD BREATH

Bad breath and a dry mouth are both symptoms of dehydration, which is caused by not drinking enough clear fluids. Try swapping a glass of refreshing water for your usual tea or coffee.

743 FILTER IN FLUORIDE

Fluoride is essential for healthy teeth, but some mineral waters contain low levels. Tap water is fortified, so make sure some of your water is filtered rather than bottled.

744 BE YOUR DENTIST'S FRIEND

Dentists recommend seeing a hygienist every three to six months as well as regular brushing. Make visits more often if you're diabetic, as you are more susceptible to gum disease.

745 A BRIGHT WHITE SMILE

For brighter teeth and to remove stains and plaque, wash your mouth out or brush with baking soda.

746 DON'T BE A-FRAYED TO CHANGE

Sticking with the same old frayed toothbrush could decrease your brushing effectiveness by as much as half. Change your toothbrush as soon as the bristles begin to fray.

747 BRUSH TWICE A DAY TO BANISH BAD BREATH

Studies reveal that some 25% of adults suffer from bad breath at some stage. You can avoid this problem by not only brushing your teeth at least twice a day, but also using a tongue scraper, as a significant amount of odour bacteria live on the tongue.

748 DON'T RUSH TO BRUSH

It is best to leave about half an hour between eating and brushing your teeth to allow the mouth to build up its normal levels of saliva and bacteria again, as these act as a protective barrier over the tooth and gum surface.

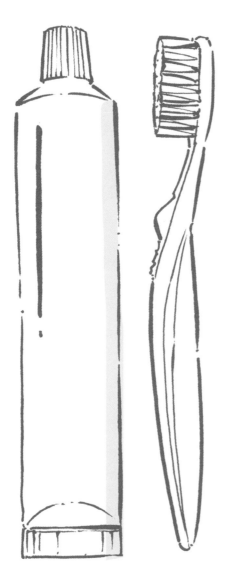

749 GIVE YOUR MOUTH A RAW DEAL

Eating raw foods increases salivation and is good for tooth health. Choose neutral carrots and celery for the best results. Citrus fruits, because they contain so much citric acid, should be accompanied by a glass of water to wash away excess acids, which could attack your teeth.

750 CHECK OUT THE CHEESEBOARD

Finishing off a meal with a piece of cheese can help protect your mouth against tooth decay, and even cooked cheese used as an ingredient in meals can help keep your teeth strong and healthy. At the end of a meal, the cheese protects dental enamel by lowering levels of mouth acidity.

MIND OVER MATTER

brainpower

751 DRINK UP TO THINK UP

The brain weighs about 1.3kg (3lb), the equivalent of a medium-sized chicken! Three-quarters of this is water, so letting yourself become dehydrated really will sap your brainpower. Aim for 1.5–2 litres (2½–3½ pints) a day.

752 EAT A BRAINY BREAKFAST

The best food to boost your brainpower at breakfast is high-fibre, carbohydrate-rich food that releases energy slowly, such as wholegrain breads and cereals, porridge or fresh fruit, plus some protein from milk, bacon, eggs or peanut butter.

753 WHIZZ UP SOME QUICK-FIX IQ FOOD

If you're feeling sluggish, whizz up a quick-fix brain boost, like a thought-boosting fruit smoothie with oats or apple purée and honey, which will keep your brain firing faster for longer.

754 BANANAS ON THE BRAIN

The glucose released into the bloodstream from carbohydrates is the brain's favourite food, and the slower and steadier it's released, the better. Bananas, apples, porridge and stoneground bread are all good snacks.

755 BREATHE DEEP TO CLEAR YOUR HEAD

The brain is the body's second largest organ and uses 20% of the total oxygen pumping around your body. Make sure you feed it well with daily deep breathing exercises to boost oxygen circulation.

756 GET CREATIVE WITH CREATINE

Studies have shown that the dietary supplement creatine, used for building body muscle, could increase brainpower by maintaining a high energy flow to the brain.

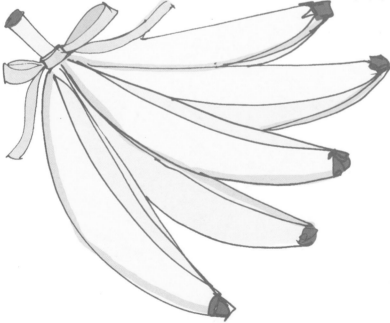

757 BE A MUSICAL GENIUS

Babies who listen to classical music have been shown to be cleverer than their peers who don't, and there is some evidence that music can help adults think clearly, too – but it's Mozart, not Motown, that brings out the brilliance!

758 BE A DOUBLE-SIDER

Try using your other hand (your left hand if you're right-handed or your right if you're left-handed) for activities such as writing, eating and sports. Experts say that this will stimulate parts of your brain that routine habits cannot reach.

759 EAT MORE CHOCOLATE

No, seriously! Studies have shown that dark chocolate has a protective effect on the brain. Combine this with trying new activities or hobbies – for example, bake your own chocolate recipes for extra mental stimulation.

760 IRON OUT MEMORY PROBLEMS

A deficiency of iron in the body will impair learning and memory skills along with cell growth in the rest of the body. To counter this, stock up on leafy green vegetables, figs, raisins, peas and meat, which contain high levels of the mineral.

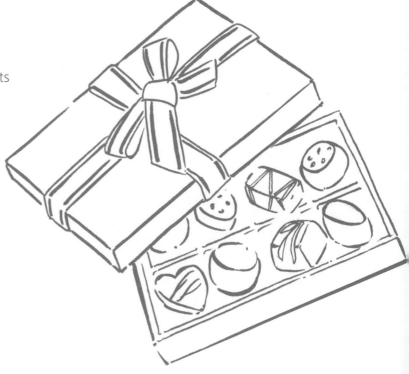

761 BE A PILLOW LOVER

Sleep allows your brain to regenerate, keeping you clear-headed and bright throughout the following day. Experts think that between seven and eight hours a night is best for optimal brainpower.

762 GET FIT TO THINK

Approximately 750ml (1¼ pints) of blood pumps through your brain every minute of the day and night, and you can boost your potential brainpower simply by increasing the efficiency of your heart by introducing a 30-minute exercise programme into your routine three times a week.

763 BE A PROTEIN PRO

Proteins are essential building blocks for the brain to make neurotransmitters, which are crucial for all thought processes. Optimize feelings of alertness by eating meat, fish, peas, beans, lentils, soya beans and soya bean products, eggs or a range of dairy products.

764 DO SOME OLIVE GOOD THINKING

Both memory and concentration are better in people whose diets include high levels of monounsaturated fats, such as those that are to be found in olive and flaxseed oils. This is because of the beneficial effect these healthy fats have on the structure of brain-cell membranes.

765 BREAKFAST LIKE A KING

People who have a proper meal at breakfast tend to have better reaction times, problem-solving abilities and a more acute memory than people who skip, skimp on or rush through their first meal of the day. So make time to breakfast royally.

766 BE AN ALL-DAY GRAZER

The brain needs nourishment 24 hours a day as it cannot store significant reserves of energy to keep it working. Missing a meal is detrimental to your thought processes, so aim to eat little and often to keep the brain's energy levels topped up.

767 GIVE YOUR BRAIN A WORKOUT

Each day, pick an object and study it for several minutes, then shut your eyes and recreate the image. Remember as much as you can, then open your eyes and see how much you missed. Repeat with different objects daily to boost concentration.

768 SHUN FAT TO STAY SHARP

High intakes of saturated fat could put people at greater risk of cognitive impairment. The healthiest diets for sharp brains are those containing oily fish like salmon and mackerel, which not only prevent degeneration of mental faculties but actually boost brainpower too.

769 BE BERRY CLEVER

A cup of blueberries a day could improve short-term memory by protecting against age-related mental decline.

770 SANDWICH SOME REST TIME

Carbohydrate foods, including starchy vegetables, pasta, potato, cereals and bread, stimulate the release of the relaxation chemical serotonin in the brain, which enables your brain to wind down after a long day.

771 GO MENTAL WITH MINERALS

Both sodium and potassium are vital ingredients when it comes to the optimal functioning of the brain, enhancing connections between neurons. Bananas are a tasty snack and high in potassium, while sodium is readily found in salt, meat and many other foods.

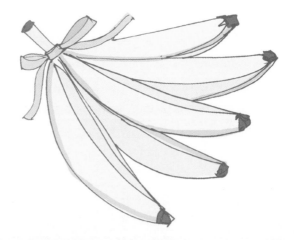

772 GET A MEATY REMINDER

Foods that are rich in protein, such as meat, fish, cheese, soya products and nuts, help the brain create dopamine, which is an essential chemical for quick thinking. Eating 75g–125g (3oz–4oz) of protein should help make you more alert and energized.

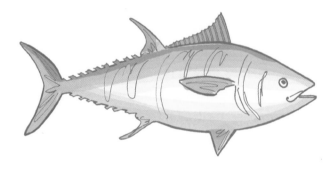

773 FISH FOR MEMORIES

Shellfish contain zinc, which boosts short-term memory and recall as well as enhances verbal and visual memory. Zinc is also found in beans, dark turkey meat and peas.

774 GET A BEANY BRAIN

Beans, peas, apples and pears contain high levels of boron, which helps enhance alertness and memory power.

775 NIBBLE NUTS FOR MEMORY

Nuts – particularly walnuts and brazil nuts – are full of the memory-boosting substance magnesium, which can improve brain function and alertness.

776 GO SLOW FOR QUICK THINKING

Low-density carbohydrate vegetables such as broccoli, spinach and pak choi, fresh herbs and low-glycaemic fruits like berries and melons release sugars slowly and help the brain work hard all day.

777 MAKE MINE AN ESPRESSO

Caffeine may improve memory by making existing brain cells swell and new ones grow, but too much can cause attention problems, so stick to espresso, which has less caffeine per serving than other coffees.

778 CHOOSE CHEESE FOR A CHAMPION BRAIN

Cheese can help to increase levels of the neurotransmitter acetylcholine in the brain, which assists general functioning. Other foods you can eat that do the same job include liver, fish, milk, broccoli, cabbage and cauliflower.

779 DRINK YOURSELF CLEVER

Your brain circuitry needs to be fully hydrated in order to function at its optimum levels, so drinking eight glasses of water a day is an essential requirement for concentration and mental alertness.

780 EAT SMALL FOR BIG SUCCESS

After a big meal, most of the body's oxygen is taken up by the intestines as they deal with the process of digestion, which means the brain gets less. This is why you often feel sleepy after a blow-out business lunch. If you want to stay alert to clinch that deal, eat light at lunch.

781 ADDRESS STRESS TO GET AHEAD

Stress hormones like cortisol destroy brain cells, which means the more stressed you are, the fuzzier your head will be. Allowing yourself to relax will help you concentrate.

782 BECOME SOYA CLEVER

Soya and soya products contain high levels of lecithin, which is essential for forming the structures of the brain, so make sure you include them in your diet.

783 RISE TO THE CHALLENGE

Challenging normal routines occasionally, like enrolling on a new course or feeling your way around your bedroom with your eyes shut, improves reaction times by forcing the brain to work harder.

784 TAKE A BREAK TO GET A BRAINWAVE

Concentrating on something for long periods of time might not be the best way to solve problems. Instead, give yourself a break to allow ideas to incubate.

785 STIMULATE YOUR SENSES

By stimulating more than one sense at once in unusual ways – for example, by sniffing vanilla essence while listening to orchestral music – you can force your brain to create new connections, thus building up your thinking potential.

786 DON'T SAY NO

Your brain does not understand negatives, so telling yourself not to think about something simply will not work. Instead, distract yourself by concentrating fully on something else and you will find that the worrying thought disappears.

787 GIVE YOURSELF A VEGETARIAN BRAIN BOOST

Vegetarians needing a brain boost could get instant benefits by upping the levels of protein (from nuts and soya) in their food or by taking a protein supplement, both of which will help stimulate the flow of blood to the brain.

788 DITCH THE CALCULATOR

Using a calculator to save time could be a false economy. It's much more beneficial for your brain if you do the maths in your head instead.

789 REMEMBER TO ADD GARLIC

Garlic has been shown to improve spatial memory and to help protect against age-related memory loss. Use it in sauces, Italian-style meals and stir fries.

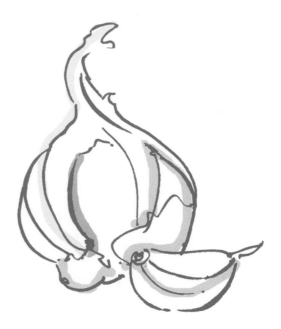

confidence

780 MAKE AN ENTRANCE

First impressions do count, so every time you walk into a room, hold your head up and your shoulders down and back. This will make you appear more confident – and if you *look* more confident, you will *be* more confident.

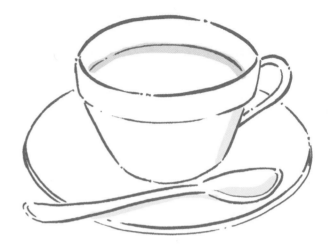

781 BE YOUR OWN HERO

If you feel your confidence slipping at a business meeting or in a social situation, just think of someone you respect and admire and spend a few minutes acting like them. Eventually it will become second nature and their self-assurance will become part of your own.

782 STAND UP TO FEEL OUTSTANDING

Standing up straight encourages you to breathe more deeply, which will in turn reduce anxiety levels and help you feel more confident.

783 CALM DOWN WITH VALERIAN

The herb valerian has been shown to help more than two-thirds of people with anxiety. Make tea infusions from roots or take supplements when you feel low.

784 LEARN TO LOVE YOURSELF

Make a list of at least five to ten things you like about yourself and carry the list around with you so you can refer to it when your self-image is low.

795 CURTAIL THE CAFFEINE

Caffeine increases heart rate, which can increase nervousness and anxiety. If you want to feel cool, calm and collected, opt for water or herbal tea instead.

796 NEGATE NERVES WITH A SNACK

If you feel sick with nerves, it could be because your stomach is empty. Confidence levels drop when we're in need of food, so have a healthy snack even if you think you're not hungry.

797 SALUTE THE SUN

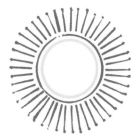

Sunlight boosts the body's natural levels of mood-boosting serotonin, so if you're feeling low on confidence a breath of fresh air could be just what you need.

798 ACCENTUATE THE POSITIVE

The next time you catch yourself having a negative thought, however small, make an effort to turn it into a positive one. Negative thinking is a bad habit that needs to be broken, and conquering the small negatives is the best way to do it.

799 LEARN TO TAKE A COMPLIMENT

People with low self-confidence often find it difficult to accept a compliment, so the next time someone says something nice about you, make an effort to listen and then thank them.

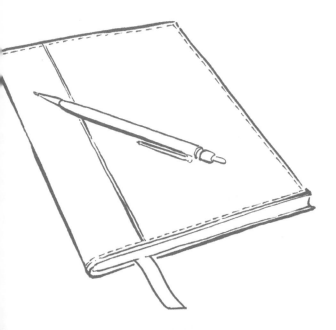

800 BE GENEROUS WITH PRAISE

Learn to pay others compliments. Giving a genuine compliment not only makes someone else feel better but can bolster your self-esteem. Look for the good in someone and tell them what you've found.

801 PAY IT FORWARD

Doing something nice for someone else has been shown to make people feel more confident, probably because it stops them thinking about themselves and focuses their attention on the positive.

depression

802 MEDITATE YOUR MOOD AWAY

Meditation can help alleviate depression by relaxing the body and reducing anxiety levels, especially if performed with breathing exercises. Aim for at least ten minutes a day for maximum benefits.

803 SAY A LITTLE PRAYER

Researchers have found that people who are religious or have religious beliefs recover faster from bouts of depression than non-religious people, so praying might help.

804 DANCE OUT OF DEPRESSION

Dance and music have been shown to help lift depression – the perfect excuse to stick on a favourite CD and start to boogie, enroll in a dance class, play the piano or sing your heart out.

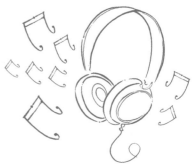

805 GET HAPPY WITH HERBS

As well as having an anti-depressant effect, St John's Wort also has antiviral and antifungal properties. It comes in tablet or infusion form and is best taken first thing in the morning.

806 LOOK ON THE SUNNY SIDE

Giving yourself a good dose of sunlight is imperative to help fight off the effects of depression, especially in the winter months, when natural daylight is in short supply. Place your desk beside a window and try to spend at least ten minutes outside at midday. If the sun is strong, however, make sure you protect your skin from the damaging effects of UV radiation.

807 PUT A FINGER ON DEPRESSION

People who have ring fingers that are longer than their index fingers are more likely to suffer from depression than others, possibly as a result of altered hormone levels in their early development.

808 GO GREEN TO FIGHT FATIGUE

Green vegetables like spinach, broccoli and kale contain high levels of B vitamins, which have been shown to help fight off depression in some sufferers by boosting general mood and alleviating fatigue.

809 BREATHE BERGAMOT TO FEEL BRIGHTER

For an instant mood boost, slip a few drops of bergamot essential oil into your bath or an essential oil burner. Be careful if it's sunny, however, as bergamot can increase sensitivity to sunlight.

810 BOOST FOLATE TO FIGHT THE BLUES

Folic acid, found in fruit, vegetables, fortified cereals and many over-the-counter supplements, has been shown to boost mood. In studies, people with lower folate levels in their blood were more likely to suffer from depression.

811 TALK YOURSELF INTO HAPPINESS

Talking to yourself can not only help ease depression but also boost self-confidence and increase the number of positive thoughts you have. Record yourself on tape talking about what you have achieved and how lucky you are, then play it back when you're feeling down.

happiness

812 FEED ON FEEL-GOOD FRUIT

Fruits containing high levels of vitamin C, like oranges, blackcurrants and kiwi fruit, can improve mood by encouraging your body to produce feel-good endorphins.

813 TRUST YOUR INSTINCTS

Women have known for years that gut reactions can often lead them on the right path, and now scientists have shown there is such a thing as a sixth sense, particularly in dangerous or risky situations. Learn to trust your woman's intuition.

814 PHONE A FRIEND TO STAY HAPPY

Research shows that people with a wide circle of friends are happier and have better self-esteem than loners. Next time you have a spare five minutes, call someone for a quick chat.

815 GET IN THE SWIM OF THINGS

Swimming is not only great exercise, but the fact that you're immersed in water means you'll also get some extra emotional benefits, as studies suggest that water can be a real mood-booster as well as a stress-releaser.

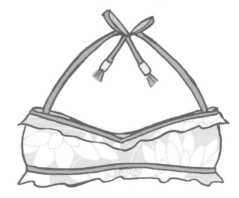

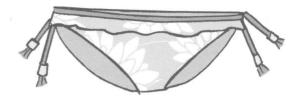

816 GET A PET

Owning a pet can boost your mood by channelling stress away and giving you a focus apart from your troubles. Don't think just traditional fur – fish and insects make good pets, too.

817 WORK OUT THOSE WORRIES

Not only is it excellent for your body, exercise is also good for your mind, stimulating the release of endorphins, which are the natural hormones for producing a feeling of happiness.

818 SMILE AWAY YOUR PROBLEMS

A simple smile lifts face muscles, releases tension in the neck, cheeks, forehead and eyebrows, and makes you feel better.

819 ADD SUNSHINE TO YOUR LIFE

Natural sunlight stimulates the body to produce vitamin D, an essential ingredient for the brain to create feel-good chemicals that can promote happiness.

820 KEEP YOUR COOL

Over a period of time, stress caused by anger can increase the risk of succumbing to heart disease and stroke by up to three times. So instead of blowing up, why not take a few deep breaths and ask yourself if it's really worth it?

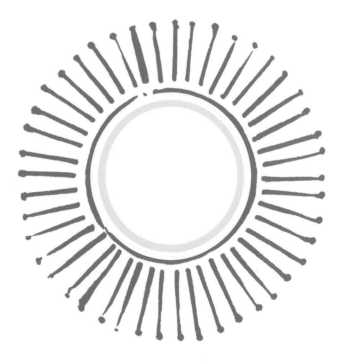

821 THINK YOURSELF HAPPY

It might be hard to believe, but brain scans have revealed that simply imagining something provokes activity in the very parts of the brain that would have been active if you were having the real experience. This suggests that thinking yourself into happy situations could actually make you happier.

822 SLEEP AWAY SADNESS

People who don't get enough sleep are less likely to be happy than their bedhead counterparts. Experts believe that seven or eight hours of sleep a night are essential if you want to wake up smiling.

823 MISS THE MIRROR

Hung up about your looks? It's not how you look that matters, say the experts, it's how you feel inside. Avoid obsessive mirror-hogging and get outside into the fresh air for an invigorating walk. It's guaranteed to make you feel a lot better.

motivation

824 DO IT IN INTERVALS

If you struggle mentally to keep going during your workout, you might want to switch to interval training instead. Using this method, your brain may respond better to short bursts of activity, so enabling you to work harder for longer.

825 DRINK UP ENERGY

Fatigue during exercise could be mostly due to dehydration, which causes the body to slow down in order to preserve essential fluids. Make sure you sip regularly to stay well hydrated.

826 THINK HAPPY FOR HEALTH

People who are happy and relaxed find it much easier to summon up motivation for things they don't want to do. Try to plan a time to do boring jobs and reward yourself when you finish – that way they won't take over your life.

827 GIVE YOURSELF GOALS

Setting yourself achievable goals to aim for throughout the day will help your body enter a natural cycle of effort and reward. Remember to reward yourself by allowing yourself a few minutes off every time you achieve something, rather than rushing on to the next task.

828 SEE YOURSELF SUCCEEDING

Visualizing yourself achieving something you want could actually help you achieve it. This is because you are moving the thought patterns in your brain away from negative thoughts towards positive, productive action.

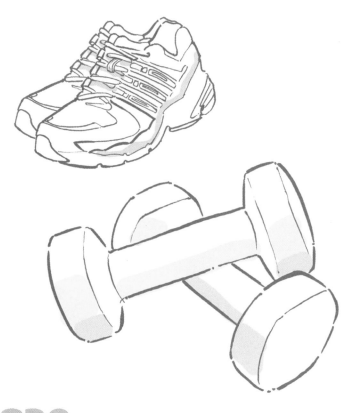

829 TREAT YOURSELF

You can train yourself to be motivated in the same way that you train a dog or teach a child – by using rewards. Allow yourself treats when you achieve something and you'll soon race through that 'to do' list.

830 BUDDY UP TO WORK HARDER

Finding a friend or gym buddy to work out with could increase your productivity by up to a third. Gym buddies help each other by making workouts fun and diverting attention away from the fact that exercise routines are often boring and repetitive.

831 MIX IT UP

No one said you had to walk the exact same route each morning or cycle the same roads day in, day out. Keep things varied and don't get stuck in a routine. You'll find that you'll look forward to the changes in scenery and varieties of activity.

832 SET REALISTIC GOALS

Set goals you know you can follow through with. Choose activities you know you can do and do well. If you find yourself constantly frustrated with your workout, for example, it could be that it's time to rework your strategy and find a better fit.

833 DRESSED FOR SUCCESS

If you look good, the chances are that you'll feel good, too. If you're feeling low, make an effort to dress up and make yourself look good, then look in the mirror and smile. You'll be amazed how much better you feel.

834 PUT IT IN WRITING

Keeping a log – of whatever it is you're trying to improve on – will help you see how well you're doing and guide you in setting new goals. If you feel you're 'stuck in a rut', set a new challenge and track your progress. Having some 'homework' could make you more diligent.

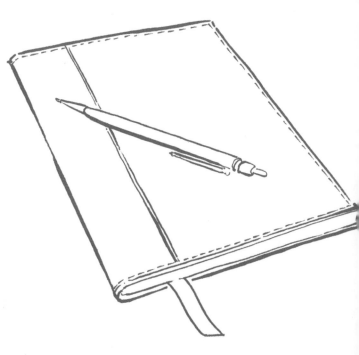

835 GIVE THE GYM A BREAK

Being active still counts as exercise, even if it's not strictly a proper workout. If you're bored with the regime at the gym, take a break. Designate an 'active' day when you don't go to the gym but make a conscious effort to exert energy in other ways. You will feel good for being active, and will have given yourself a break from your normal routine.

836 BOOGIE ON DOWN

Playing your favourite music or a selection of uplifting, inspiring songs while you work out or do unpleasant tasks has been shown in studies to increase enjoyment and motivation. Grab that broom and don't be afraid to dance around the kitchen while you clean!

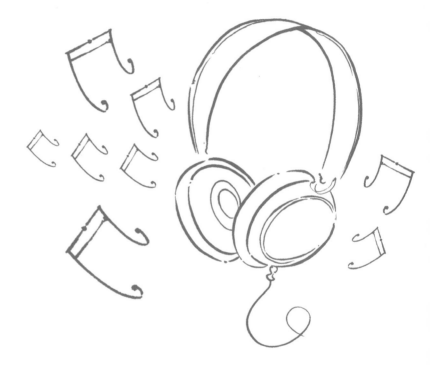

negative thoughts

837 THINK POSITIVE TO STAY PAIN-FREE

Negative thoughts not only make you feel bad but also increase the perception of pain. People who are inclined to think negatively about things perceive more pain than those with a tendency towards a more positive frame of mind.

838 LOCK AWAY NEGATIVITY

Start keeping a negative notebook in which to lock away destructive thoughts. Every time you think negatively, write the thought down in the notebook and leave it there so the notebook gets filled up, instead of your brain.

839 ATTEND TO THE DETAILS

People who are in the habit of over-generalizing are more likely to have negative thoughts than those who pay attention to the details. So the next time you feel low, instead of just accepting it, think about why you feel bad and try to do something about it.

840 MAKE A THOUGHT CHAIN

Carry around a pocketful of paperclips and every time you have a negative thought about yourself, simply hook another paperclip onto the chain. At the end of the day, you might well be amazed to discover just how negative you are. Once you've identified your negative triggers, work at transforming them into positive ones.

841 BE A CONTROL FREAK

Instead of worrying about things you can't change, concentrate on the things you can change and control – that way you'll feel you're achieving something.

842 A THOUGHT FOR THE DAY

Start every day with a positive thought about yourself. It could be something you like or enjoy doing, or something you feel – just as long as it's positive.

843 BREATHE DEEPLY TO STOP THE DOWNWARD SPIRAL

If you feel negative thoughts beginning to overwhelm you, stop and take a deep breath. The idea here is that negative thinking is linked to the stress response, which can be halted by a series of long, slow, deep breaths.

844 LISTEN FOR THE GOOD THINGS

The next time you feel defensive about something someone has said, think about the comment again before you react. Then, instead of taking it as criticism, try to extract positives from it.

845 DON'T SPEAK OUT OF TURN

Listen to the way you say things, particularly to those you love the most. Do you say what you mean or do the words come out in a critical way? Often people can seem to be criticizing without meaning to. Think positively about other people, and make sure they know it.

187

relaxation

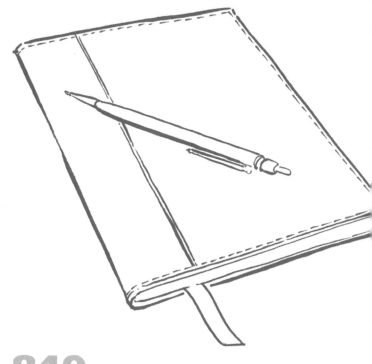

846 IT'S GOOD TO TALK

Talking has been shown to help relaxation by allowing the brain to work around problems, encouraging other points of view and reducing anxiety and tension. Next time you feel stressed, tell someone.

847 MAKE A LIST TO LIKE YOURSELF

If you're feeling stressed or tense, take a few minutes off to make a list of five things you can do well and five things you really like about yourself. Then look at it next time you feel anxious to help you relax.

848 ENDORPHIN ENDOWMENT

Exercise releases natural chemicals in your body, called endorphins, that actually alter your mood and make you feel better. Aim for at least 30 minutes, three or four times a week, preferably out in the fresh air.

849 TAKE THREE DEEP BREATHS

Put one hand on your chest and the other on your stomach. Take a deep breath in and feel the hand on your stomach move but the hand on your chest remain still. Exhale and then take a deep breath in and hold it for a count of three. Exhale through your mouth and count to five before taking the next deep breath.

850 CREATE A CUNNING PLAN

Write down your goals for next week, next month or next summer. Write down three things you can do that will help you reach each of your future targets, then work at achieving them.

851 DO SOMETHING DIFFERENT

A new challenge is a great way to promote relaxation. It could be something simple, such as reading a new type of book or rearranging your desk, or something major, such as going on holiday or joining a club.

852 MEDITATE TO SEND PROBLEMS PACKING

Meditation can help people suffering from chronic diseases as well as stress-related disorders, including abdominal pain, stomach ulcers and chronic diarrhoea. Meditation helps slow the breathing rate and increases oxygen consumption and blood flow to the brain, which produces a more relaxed brainwave rhythm.

853 LEND A HELPING HAND

One of the best ways to help you destress your life and start to relax is to take the time to help somebody else. Take care of a neighbour's garden or mow their lawn, for example, or volunteer some of your spare time at a nursing home or a shelter for abandoned animals.

854 LAUGH AT YOURSELF

Although it's hard to do, studies have shown that laughing at yourself is a great way to release inner tension and improve your outlook on life. Instead of worrying or becoming tense or angry, try to make a point of seeing the funny side of events.

855 BREAK OFF AND BREATHE

Focusing on your breathing every now and then is a simple yet brilliant way to help you relax. Wherever you are, you can take a few minutes out to do some deep breathing. Do this a few times and you will soon feel your body relax.

856 GET A FURRY FRIEND

Keeping a pet helps people relax, stop worrying and maintain a positive outlook on life.

857 ALL-OVER MUSCLE RELAXATION

Starting with your toes, tighten the muscles until they start to ache. Then completely relax, letting the toes go limp. Repeat this with all the major muscle groups – legs, arms, shoulders, neck – then the hands. Learn the difference between tense and relaxed, and when you feel tense, do a body check to see which muscles need relaxing.

858 A WORD IN YOUR EAR

Choose a word you like, close your eyes and concentrate on it, repeating it over and over again in your head. Studies have shown that this one-word relaxation technique could deliver fantastic mind and body benefits, reducing stress and promoting relaxation.

859 TAKE TIME TO STAY CALM

Daily meditation has been shown to reduce stress levels and boost your body's immunity, so spend a couple of minutes meditating every morning, concentrating on breathing and emptying your mind of extraneous thoughts.

860 FINISH IT OFF

The way our brains are designed, they continue to hang on to a thought until it's finished, which means the most stressful situation is one where you're surrounded by lots of unfinished tasks. The best way to relax is by finishing things one at a time.

861 TUNE IN FOR A RELAXING MINI-BREAK

Take some time out every day and listen to relaxing music like classical, soft piano, repetitive harmonics or strings. As you listen, let your mind empty itself of all thoughts to help you relax.

862 TAKE A GOOD LOOK AT YOURSELF

Sitting in front of a mirror and doing some deep breathing for five minutes could help you unwind and relax. You'll be able to spot signs of stress, such as hunched shoulders or a tightly closed mouth, and then relax them away.

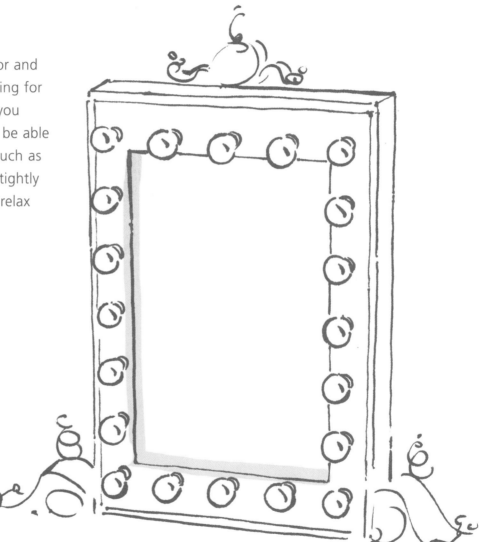

seasonal affective disorder

863 WATCH OUT FOR WINTER BLUES

Seasonal affective disorder (SAD) can manifest itself in feeling low, anxiety, fatigue, weight gain, carbohydrate craving, lack of energy and difficulty concentrating during dark winter months. Slight depression isn't the same thing.

864 FLY OFF TO FREEDOM

Taking a holiday abroad at the darkest time of the year could be the key to alleviating SAD. Just a week of sunlight can stave off symptoms for up to a month afterwards.

865 HAPPINESS IN A BOX

Exposure to light boxes has been found to help sufferers of SAD by safely mimicking the effects of summer sun.

866 CHOOSE PROTEIN TO BOOST YOUR MOOD

To avoid blood sugar surges, which can affect mood, stick to protein-rich foods that release sugar slowly – such as turkey, chicken, salmon, kidney beans or lentils – or slow-release complex carbohydrates like wholemeal bread and brown rice.

867 RELAX TO STAY HAPPY

Relaxation therapies, such as Tai Chi, meditation, yoga and massage have been shown to reduce the symptoms of SAD. So next time you feel like you are suffering, get yourself to a class – a deep relaxation treat and being around others may help.

868 D FOR DEPRESSION

In a trial, SAD sufferers who took 400 IU (international units) of vitamin D a day during the winter felt more enthusiastic, inspired and alert, probably because the vitamin raises levels of the mood-lifting brain chemical serotonin.

869 WALK IT OUT

Getting outside for a 15-minute walk every day can help relieve SAD because sunlight enables the body to produce vitamin D, raising mood-boosting brain chemicals and aiding circulation.

870 HERBAL HIGH

The mood-boosting effects of the herb St John's Wort were marked in almost half of those who took it in one study. It can have side effects, so check with your doctor before taking it.

871 TIME OF THE MONTH?

If you find your PMS (PMT) symptoms get worse during the winter months, it could be a sign of SAD. Exercise and spending more time outside in the natural light should help alleviate symptoms.

872 PARTY ON

If you're suffering from SAD, the last thing you want to do is go out and party the night away, but it could really be the best thing for you. Studies have shown that people who make themselves socialize when they're low feel happier sooner than stay-at-home hermits.

873 GET ON YOUR BIKE

Regular exercise – inside or outside – could be almost as effective as light therapy for sufferers of the winter blues, probably because of the mood-boosting endorphins that are released into the body following any type of strenuous exercise.

stress

874 SING IT OUT

The next time you notice the symptoms of stress and feel like shouting with frustration, sing your favourite song. The words will make you feel happier and singing will regulate your breathing, thus reducing the body's stress response.

875 SLEEP YOUR WAY THROUGH STRESS

Stress can cause sleep problems, leaving you fatigued and vulnerable to illness and increasing anxiety, nervousness and irritability. If you find yourself overwhelmed by worries, write them down, which will help you forget them until morning.

876 WORK OUT YOUR PERSONALITY TYPE

Type A personalities, who are more likely to be perfectionist, controlling, pessimistic, inflexible, and frightened of change than others, are more likely to suffer stress. If this sounds like you, you could be in need of stress relief. Combating it early could stop you suffering ill-effects.

877 DON'T STRESS WITH ESPRESSOS

Beware of reaching for a cup of coffee in an attempt to reduce feelings of stress. Coffee raises adrenaline levels by more than a third to make you feel more stressed, especially if you drink it alone. Instead, opt for herbal tea or a glass of water to soothe your nerves.

878 SNIFF STRESS AWAY

Several essential oils have powerful calming effects. Keep a bottle of lavender, sandalwood or camomile oil to hand and sniff as needed. Or dab a few drops of the oils on a hanky and carry it with you.

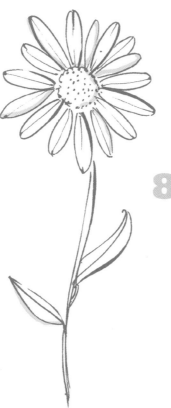

879 DON'T LET STRESS AFFECT YOUR JOB

Not only can stress adversely affect your concentration, making you perform poorly at college or on the job, but the hormones it releases into your body can cause weight gain or weight loss.

880 FLEX YOUR FACE

Studies have shown that many women react to tension by clenching the jaw, which only makes stress worse. If you find yourself with a clenched jaw, stretch your facial muscles by opening your mouth and eyes in a look of surprise. Hold this expression for a few seconds before relaxing.

881 BREATHE AWAY PANIC

Lie on your back and balance a book on your belly, then breathe in. The book should rise up. Now that you know what belly breathing feels like, practise it to slow yourself down, regulate breathing and avoid hyperventilation. It is a good remedy forpanic attacks and stress.

ageing

882 BE A HONEY IF YOU WANT TO STAY SHARP

Too much sugar in the diet has been found to leave damaging beta amyloid deposits in the brain, which can contribute to brain degeneration and Alzheimer's disease. Swap sugar for healthier alternatives like honey or maple syrup.

883 COP YOURSELF A FEW EXTRA YEARS

Recent studies have shown that copper is essential for reducing age-related disintegration of body tissues. Get your doses from oysters, crab, nuts, soya beans, wholegrains, peas and lentils.

884 WORK OUT TO WARD OFF DISEASE

Studies have shown that regular exercise boosts the levels of white blood cells in the blood. These white cells are responsible for fighting illnesses from flu to cancer and preventing tissue degeneration, so regular exercise really could help you fight ageing.

885 DON'T BE FAZED, TAKE EFAS

Essential fatty acids (EFAs), found in oily fish, walnuts and oils such as olive, sunflower, linseed (flaxseed) and evening primrose, reduce inflammatory chemicals in the body and lead to better mental health and clarity. To keep your wits about you as you grow old, make sure you have some every day.

886 BONE UP ON CHEESE

The calcium in cheese, particularly full-fat cheese, is essential for preventing the bone-thinning disease osteoporosis. Experts say that having three small portions of dairy products a day can help maintain strong bones.

887 REMEMBER YOUR GLASSES

As we get older our sensitivity to thirst decreases, leading to dehydration and possible health problems. So it's even more important for older people to make sure they drink at least eight caffeine-free, non-alcoholic drinks a day.

888 MUNCH DOWN YOUR BLOOD PRESSURE

Eggs, wheat, kidney, soya, alfalfa and rice bran all contain high levels of the vitamin-like substance coenzyme Q10, which is thought to boost immunity, lower blood pressure, prevent heart attacks and reduce the symptoms of ageing.

889 POWER UP YOUR MEMORY

Gingko biloba, a tree extract that has been used by the Chinese for about 2,800 years, improves mental function by soaking up harmful free radicals and improving neurotransmission within the brain, promoting good blood circulation and enhancing memory.

890 WORK AWAY JOINT PAIN

Strengthening your muscles with regular exercise could help prevent or end pain from joints and bone degeneration in later life. A tiny increase in thigh strength could reduce risk of knee osteoarthritis by up to a third.

891 MAKE EVERY DAY A D-DAY

Experts say vitamin D is essential for the body to absorb enough calcium to keep bones healthy and strong. The vitamin is converted in the body on contact with sunlight, so make sure you get outside for some fresh air every day as you get older.

892 WALK THE WALK

Walking improves circulation, bone strength and immune functions and can help people look between five and eight years younger in middle and later life. Half an hour a day is ideal.

893 BE A SUPERBRAN

Fibre has been shown to be important in preventing constipation and helping lower cholesterol. It also protects against colon cancer and helps regulate blood sugar.

894 FOLLOW THE RULER

The falling ruler test measures reaction time, which deteriorates with age. Ask someone to hold a wooden ruler by the top, large numbers – 45cm (18in) – down, suspended centred above your thumb and middle finger. Have them drop the ruler without warning three times, while you try to catch it, then average your score. The 28cm (11in) mark is normal for a 20-year-old and 15cm (6in) for a 60-year-old.

895 KEEP LIGHT TO STAY BRIGHT

After the age of 65, overweight people have a higher chance of a decrease in mental function than people of normal or lower weight, so it's important to stay slender.

bad habits

896 UNEARTH HIDDEN DIET HORRORS

Write down everything you eat for three days. Do you add a lot of butter, sauces or salad dressings? Rather than eliminating these foods, cut back your portions.

897 JUMP FOR BETTER JOINTS

Get into the high-impact habit. Studies have shown that to keep muscles and bones strong, resistance training that involves impact, such as running, walking, skipping rope and weight training, can be more beneficial than smooth, slow movements like swimming and cycling.

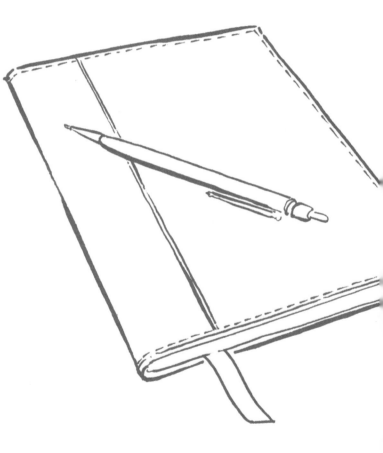

898 FENG SHUI YOUR BAD HABITS AWAY

According to feng shui practitioners, bad habits could be due to problems in the bedroom health area. Draw a plan of your room with the main entrance at the bottom and divide it into nine roughly equal squares. Your health area is the middle square on the left. Make sure it is clutter free or fill it with round-leaved plants.

899 GIVE IN TO CHOCOLATE

Chocolate – especially dark chocolate – can boost your mood by increasing levels of the amino acid L-tryptophan, which encourages feel-good serotonin to be released, so don't feel guilty about tucking in.

900 WRITE IT DOWN

Size up your bad habits by listing all the pros and cons. Having a clear list of good and bad points to compare makes it far easier to measure up the benefits of giving up a bad habit. Look at the list every time you feel your motivation slipping.

901 STOP LATE-NIGHT SNACKING

Eating a big meal at night, or snacking through the evening, impairs sleep quality by sending your body mixed messages and giving it heavy work to do, making it more difficult for you to get to sleep. Instead, eat earlier in the evening.

902 DO IT TODAY

Procrastinating – putting everything off until tomorrow – not only reduces your efficiency but also causes stress. The longer you hold 'to do' lists in your head, the more stressful they become. Vow to do one chore every day.

903 DON'T BE PICKY

Rather than eliminating the problem, picking spots can introduce dirt and bacteria onto the skin surface, increasing chances of infection, not to mention the effects of redness and scarring. So, for healthier skin, don't pick – cover up blemishes instead.

904 CULL YOUR CRAVINGS CULPRITS

Foods you crave and eat the most may be causing a lot of your health problems, say researchers who are worried about people becoming dependent on sugar highs from snack foods. Chief culprits to cut are pastry, cakes, biscuits (cookies) and doughnuts.

905 WALK OFF THE WEIGHT

If you're a couch potato and don't spend much time outside, make yourself walk in the fresh air for at least ten minutes a day. Not only will it boost your metabolism and help stretch out muscles, the natural light will raise vitamin D levels.

906 CUT CAFFEINE TO STOP STRESS

Coffee drinkers can have up to a third more stress hormones circulating in their system than non-coffee drinkers, making them more prone to stress. Aim for no more than three cups a day, swapping the rest for water or herbal teas.

907 SET AN ALARM TO CRACK THE CRAVING

If you get a craving for a bad habit – like smoking or filling up on cakes or ice cream – set a timer for five minutes, then see if you still have the craving when it goes off. Experts believe this time lapse can cure cravings.

908 TAKE A BREAK AT WORK

Far from being efficient, workaholics who don't take breaks during the day are up to a quarter less efficient than those with healthier working practices. Working through breaks is a false economy, so make yourself have at least three breaks – when you DON'T think about work at all.

909 KEEP HUNGER IN THE CAN

Downing a carbonated drink at breakfast is likely to make you more hungry at lunchtime, even if it's one of the sugar-free varieties. Don't start your day with the fizz.

910 EAT EARLY TO STAY SLIM

Recent research studies have shown that people who regularly eat breakfast consume more vitamins and minerals throughout the day than those who skip breakfast, and they are also less likely to be overweight.

911 SWITCH SWEETS FOR FRUIT

If you find yourself munching on high-sugar, high-calorie sweets for a treat, try switching to chopped fruit or no-sugar yogurt instead. Both of these are sweet but healthy, natural alternatives.

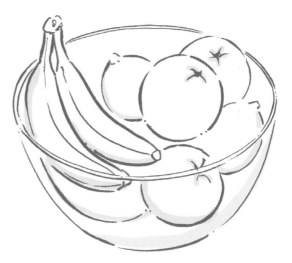

912 BE A HUNGER MONGER

Instead of scoffing food whenever you get the opportunity, think about eating moderately and according to your natural appetite instead. To do this, rate your hunger on a scale from one (absolutely starving) to ten (completely stuffed). Then, only start eating at two or three and finish at seven.

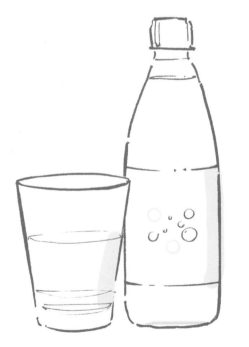

climate changes

913 COTTON ON

During high-heat, high-humidity periods, it's easier to develop the yeast infection candida. Opting for cotton underwear can help prevent problems arising, as can loose trousers and skirts.

914 STAY WET IN WINTER

Water is important all year round but in winter, because of central heating and lots of stress on the body as temperatures change suddenly from cold outside to hot inside, it's even more important to drink eight glasses a day.

915 RING THE WINTER CHANGES

Rings that get tighter in the winter could be a sign of fluid retention caused by too much salt, along with tighter shoes and socks that leave lines on ankles that aren't there in warmer weather. If this happens, drink more water.

916 BANISH BODY ODOUR FASHIONABLY

Sweat and underarm odour are worse in the summer because it's harder for sweat to evaporate, leaving it in contact with the body for longer. Wear loose clothes in natural materials like cotton or linen, and avoid nylon.

917 STEAM AHEAD TO BEAT WINTER COUGHS

People are more prone to developing coughs and lung problems in dry weather, which can dry out the inner membranes of the lungs and cause trauma to them. To alleviate seasonal coughs, have regular hot baths or steam inhalations.

918 CHOOSE SEASONAL FOODS

In winter, root vegetables are more nutritious because the plants push their energy reserves into the roots to avoid the cold. In summer, flowering fruits like tomatoes contain more goodness. So follow nature for the healthiest diet.

919 DON'T GET SORE, GET SCREENED

Cold sores are more common in the summer, when sudden exposure to sunlight puts the skin under stress. To avoid them, acclimatize slowly and use a sunscreen.

920 WALK YOURSELF HAPPY

Just 15 minutes of daylight a day can help prevent the winter blues by giving your body a good dose of vitamin D, so get out in the fresh air.

921 DON'T HAVE A FAT WINTER

Many people put on weight during the winter because their activity levels drop and food cravings increase with colder weather. Try indoor exercises like yoga to help you spring into spring.

922 COOL AS A CUCUMBER

Cucumbers, mung beans and watermelon are particularly good foods to eat in the summer because they help keep your body cool and aid salt balance.

923 TURN OFF WHEN YOU TURN IN

Sleep quality and quantity are both better when the bedroom temperature is on the low side, so turning off the central heating or turning down the thermostat on winter nights could help you get a better night's sleep.

924 HIBERNATE FOR BETTER IMMUNITY

Studies have shown that in winter people need more sleep than in summer to reboot their immune systems, so let yourself have an extra half an hour in bed for that all-important extra winter resistance.

925 PUT A HAT ON INFECTIONS

We lose a lot of our body heat through the skin on our head and neck, so covering up with a hat and scarf can help your body fight off infections by keeping you snug.

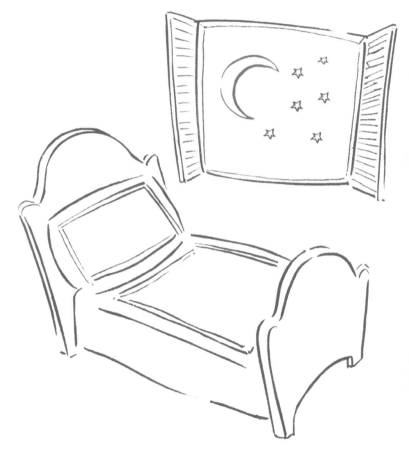

926 SEE THE LIGHT

If you find yourself craving more starchy and sugary foods during the winter months, you may be suffering from seasonal affective disorder (SAD), which can be helped by daily exposure to natural sunlight or by light-box treatment.

927 ESCAPE GERMS WITH ECHINACEA

Sudden, abrupt changes in the ambient temperature can take a toll on the body's energy levels, making it more prone to succumb to infections. If you're faced with hotter or colder climates, take echinacea, which has been shown to strengthen the immune system.

928 BREATHE EASY ALL YEAR ROUND

Spring is called the allergy season but air quality is, in fact, worse in winter than at any other time. Fight allergies by upping your intake of free-radical fighters in fresh fruit and vegetables.

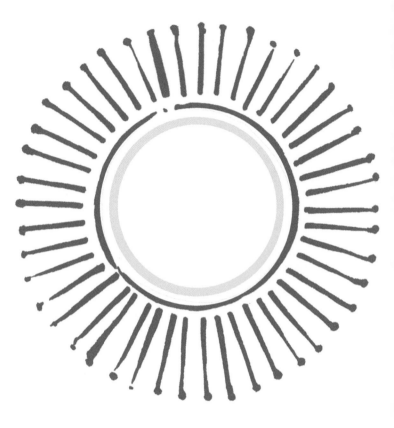

hangovers

929 PALE IS BEAUTIFUL

Recent research suggests that dark, sweet drinks like brandy, rum and whisky contain more 'congeners', which produce the effects of hangovers, than paler drinks like white wine and vodka.

930 ALTERNATE DRINKS TO AVOID A HANGOVER

Alternate alcoholic drinks with water if you want to keep yourself hangover free the next day by keeping your body hydrated and giving your liver a chance to work on excess alcohol.

931 THINK QUALITY NOT QUANTITY

Cheaper brands of drinks often contain more toxins and are therefore harder for the liver to cope with, causing worse hangovers. Go for quality rather than quantity – the expense might motivate you to limit your drinking, too.

932 BE A WATER BABY

The dehydration that alcohol causes often plays a major role in the hangover scenario. Matching alcoholic drinks glass for glass with water, and then slugging back another glass or two of water before going to bed, will help combat this.

933 DETOX WITH A BEET DRINK

For a detoxifying antidote to all that partying, try beetroot juice mixed with the juices of carrot, apple, celery and ginger. The celery contains various antioxidant compounds that will help neutralize the effects of cigarette smoke, while the ginger will help relieve any nausea, stomachache or diarrhoea.

934 HAVE HONEY TO BURN OFF ALCOHOL

Before or while you're drinking, have a large glass of grapefruit juice, and eat some honey. The grapefruit is a liver tonic, and the honey helps your body burn off alcohol in your system.

935 BOOST YOUR B INTAKE FOR BETTER MORNINGS

Take a combination of B-complex vitamins, vitamin C and zinc before a night of drinking, and then again in the morning, to help your system replace what you have lost with your overindulgence. Research shows that your system turns to B vitamins when it is under stress, and alcohol depletes levels further.

936 BARK BACK AT PAIN

Willowbark tablets are a natural alternative to over-the-counter headache pills because they contain a form of salicylate, which is the active ingredient in aspirin.

937 DON'T SOBER UP WITH A COFFEE

Drinking caffeine, which is in its highest concentrations in filter coffee, is a diuretic and will rob your body of even more water and nutrients. Try water or a sports drink instead, to replace electrolytes and give you an energy boost.

938 CALM WITH CAMOMILE

Camomile and peppermint tea are good stomach settlers if you've overindulged, while aloe vera can neutralize excess stomach acid and soothe an irritated gastrointestinal tract.

939 SPICE UP YOUR LIFE

Ginger is one of the most effective natural remedies for nausea and indigestion, stimulating metabolism to encourage the elimination of toxins.

940 FEEL FINE AND DANDELION

The herb dandelion is a traditional liver tonic that has been shown to reduce the severity and duration of headaches.

941 PRESS YOUR LUCK

Try the ancient Chinese art of acupressure to relieve morning nausea. With your thumb, apply continuous pressure to the soft area between your thumb and index finger on either hand for several minutes.

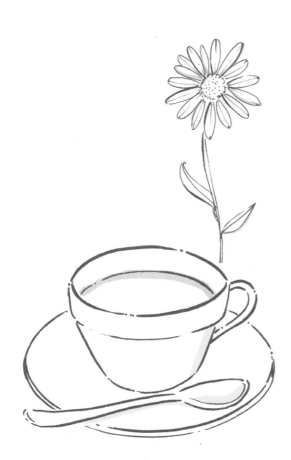

942 MILK A CURE

Milk thistle is renowned for its ability to support and stimulate the working of the liver, which is the organ primarily responsible for detoxifying alcohol within the body. Take a dose of milk thistle before you go out and one when you get back for the best results.

943 DON'T GET A RUM DEAL

Drinking rum, brandy and whisky is more likely to cause a hangover than drinking white wine, gin or vodka because they contain methanol, formaldehyde and formic acid, which are the chemicals chiefly responsible for a hangover's headache and accompanying rapid heart rate.

944 BECOME AN ICE MAIDEN

Soothe a throbbing hangover headache the natural way with an ice pack. Soak cottonwool pads in cold camomile tea and then place them on your eyelids to reduce the swelling.

945 CROSS OUT CROISSANTS

Eating a breakfast of croissants, buttery brioches or high-sugar cereals can send your blood sugar level on a rollercoaster ride of ups and downs, while fatty foods can make you feel sick. Rather than endure this, stick to healthy options like fruit and wholegrain foods.

946 REFRESH YOURSELF WITH A SEA BREEZE

Bloody Marys and Sea Breezes are two of the least toxic alcoholic drinks because the vodka they are made with doesn't contain any congeners and they contain health-giving fruit juices, too.

947 FILL UP WITH FOOD

Taking alcoholic drinks on an empty stomach brings about a drop in blood sugar that makes you feel light-headed and drunk, then keeps it low throughout the night and into the following day, resulting in a major hangover.

live long & healthy

948 BE PART OF THE CROWD

Death rates are twice as high for the most socially isolated people compared with those with strong social ties, so your friends really can help you live longer.

949 THE PEEL-GOOD FACTOR

Adding more potassium to the diet can lower blood pressure, while a diet deprived of potassium can actually raise blood pressure. Eating one banana per day provides the extra 400mg of potassium needed to slash the odds of suffering a fatal stroke by 40%.

950 GIVE YOURSELF A RAW DEAL

According to studies, if you don't consume fruit daily, your risk of stomach cancer doubles or even triples, and raw is best. Munch on raw fruit and vegetables.

951 WEAR A COPPER

Copper is an essential supplement for reducing age-related disintegration of body tissues and it is an a nonallergenic material. Many people, particularly arthritis sufferers, wear copper bracelets for the absorption of the mineral into the skin.

952 HAVE A HEARTY DOSE OF ONION

Consuming half an onion a day, or the equivalent in juice, raises HDL (good) cholesterol by an average of 30% in most people with heart disease or cholesterol problems, extending life expectancy and boosting health.

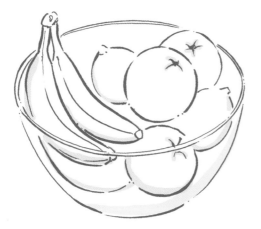

953 CURIOSITY KEEPS THE CAT ALIVE

The more curious you are, the more likely you are to live longer, say scientists who found that curious people were 30% less likely to die than people who weren't.

954 OH FOR OKINAWA

Okinawans live longer than any other race on earth. Their secrets include eating lots of soya products, stopping eating before they are completely full and daily exercise.

955 BE OPTIMISTIC

Optimists live about 20% longer than pessimists, so making yourself believe that the glass is half full rather than half empty really could enhance your health.

956 REST ASSURED

Rest is as important as exercise in helping your body stay healthy for longer. Regular exercise along with daily relaxation and at least one rest day a week may add years to the life span.

957 MAKE EACH MEAL SMALLER

People may be able to extend the length of their lives by cutting calorific intake by just 10%, as long as they aren't depriving themselves of essential nutrients as well.

958 GET SPIRITUAL

People who attend religious ceremonies regularly are likely to live significantly longer than their non-religious friends, so maybe it's time to rediscover old beliefs.

959 GO BACK TO YOUR ROOTS

People who behave as if they're younger live longer and age less quickly. You don't need to dress in the clothes you wore as a teenager, just revive a few of the things you liked doing when young.

960 PINE FOR YOUR YOUTH

Pine bark extract (pycnogenol) and grape-seed extract contain powerful antioxidants that can help your body counteract the damaging signs of ageing.

961 SAY OMM TO BEAT AGEING

Meditation reduces stress, which is one of the major causes of the ageing process, and taking up yoga and other meditative techniques in old age has been shown to enhance quality of life.

love

962 DON'T BE A PRUNE PRUDE

Not only are prunes top of the healthy, cancer-beater charts, they also have aphrodisiac properties. Eros, the Greek god of love, is said to have dipped his arrow in prune juice. You, however, can just eat them instead!

963 GET IN THE MED FOR LOVE

In the Mediterranean, pistachios and pine nuts are considered aphrodisiacs and certain spices, like cinnamon and nutmeg, are said to arouse both men and women.

964 TIE THE KNOT TO STAY ALIVE

Being married encourages healthy
behaviour. Married people are apparently
more likely to wear seat belts, be active,
eat breakfast and not smoke, so tying the
knot could help your health.

965 CHOC FULL OF DESIRE

Chocolate releases endorphins into the body that make us feel happier and more relaxed, which is why it's considered such an effective aphrodisiac. Enjoy!

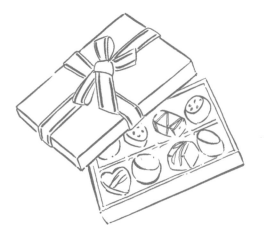

966 KISS AND MAKE UP

Arguments between couples weaken their immune system, making them more susceptible to illness. People who feel loved and supported are less likely to suffer blockages in their heart arteries than unhappy people.

sex

967 SEX IS GOOD FOR YOU

Working the muscles around your sex organs regularly keeps them strong and healthy. For men, this can help reduce the chance of suffering prostrate cancer and for women it helps prevent incontinence problems. You can safely consider your lovemaking to be a health-giving activity.

968 LIVE LONGER WITH THE BIG-O

Orgasms could help you live longer. People with an active sex life who regularly reach orgasm are half as likely to die at an earlier age than those who don't. So the older you get, the more important sex is!

969 GET SOME SATISFACTION

Sexual dissatisfaction is potentially a serious risk factor when it comes to heart attacks in women, with women who are satisfied in bed being much less likely to suffer from heart problems.

970 ZINC INTO THE MOOD

A natural aphrodisiac and fertility booster, zinc is found in pumpkin and sesame seeds, cheese, chicken and turkey, wholegrains, pine nuts, brown rice, fish and seafood. Not forgetting (surprise, surprise) oysters!

971 SAFEGUARD HIM WITH REGULAR SEX

Men who have sex every other day are significantly less likely to develop life-threatening prostate cancer than those who sow their oats less often, so upping your sexual antics could aid his health as well as yours.

972 MORNING GLORY

The male's testosterone levels have been found to drop by nearly a quarter in the mid- to late evening, so don't take it personally if he doesn't desire you before going to bed. Testosterone levels and, therefore, sex drive, are usually highest first thing in the morning.

973 TAKE TO THE FLOOR

Make your orgasms more powerful and work your pelvic floor muscles at the same time by contracting and relaxing them.

974 ENJOY SEX THROUGH THE BIG CHANGE

Women going through menopause who eat about 100g (3½oz) of tofu daily or drink one cup of soya milk receive an oestrogen boost that makes sex more satisfying and pleasurable.

975 TAKE IODINE FOR LOW SEX DRIVE

In some people, low sex drive could be due to an underactive thyroid gland, so if you seldom feel in the mood, visit your doctor to have your thyroid checked; increased iodine could be the answer.

976 THYME FOR BED

Chromium, found in thyme, and also wholegrains, meat, cheese and brewer's yeast, is thought to increase sperm count in men and sex drive in both sexes.

977 GET LIVELY WITH LIVER

Vitamins A and E are vital for the production of sex hormones, which boost sex drive. Find them in liver, dairy produce, oily fish, dark green leafy vegetables and yellow-orange fruits.

978 DON'T LET STRESS SPOIL SEX

Vitamin C and magnesium, essential for the proper functioning of sex organs, are used up in times of stress, so it's important to replenish them with foods like citrus fruits, red berries, potatoes, kiwi, chicken, tuna and green leafy vegetables.

979 TRYP THE SEX FANTASTIC

Foods containing tryptophan, such as bananas, milk, cottage cheese and turkey, not only encourage sleep but can also boost sex drive by increasing comfort sensations and reducing stress. Milk chocolate contains tryptophan, too, plus phenylethylamine, a chemical thought to be released at times of arousal.

980 BE A DOMESTIC GODDESS

Bizarre as it may sound, the smell of cinnamon buns has been shown to boost male sexual arousal. Pumpkin-pie scent was also found to be very erotic, so spending a few hours in the kitchen could pay exciting sex dividends.

981 GET HOT TO LOSE WEIGHT

Having sex burns approximately 150 calories every 30 minutes, so if you have vigorous sex for an hour you could burn about 300 calories – which is roughly equivalent to what you would burn if you went for a brisk one-hour walk. Why not try for a marathon?

982 GLOW WITH THE FLOW

Sex helps increase blood flow to your organs. As a fresh blood supply arrives, the body's cells, organs and muscles are filled with fresh oxygen and hormones; and as the used blood is removed, it takes away the waste products that are responsible for feelings of fatigue.

983 GET HEART HEALTHY IN BED

Sex helps lower cholesterol levels. More importantly, it tips the HDL/LDL (good/bad) cholesterol balance towards the healthier HDL side by promoting blood flow and increasing feelings of wellbeing.

984 USE SEX AS A STRESS BUSTER

Research studies reveal that people who have frequent, pleasurable sex handle stress better. The profound relaxation that typically follows sex, when the hormone rush causes the body to relax, may be one of the few times when people allow themselves to let go completely.

985 NATURE'S FAVOURITE PAINKILLER

Endorphins are released from the brain during lovemaking. These natural opiates act as powerful analgesics in the body, easing aches and pains.

986 MAKE HAY WITH DHEA

The natural hormone DHEA, which is produced in response to sexual excitement, helps strengthen the immune system, improves cognition, promotes bone growth, and maintains and repairs tissues in the body. It may also contribute to cardiovascular health and even function as a mild antidepressant.

987 BUILD UP BONES IN THE BOUDOIR

Regular sexual activity appears to lift levels of testosterone and oestrogen hormones, which act in the body to strengthen bones and muscles.

988 BE A HONEY IN BED

Honey contains high levels of boron, which helps the body metabolize and utilize oestrogen and enhances levels of testosterone, the hormone responsible for revving up sex drive.

travel

989 TRAVEL A LITTLE AT A TIME

Jetlag tends to be a problem if four or more time zones are crossed, and the effects are generally worse travelling eastwards rather than westwards because the body copes better with a lengthening day than with a shortening day.

980 DO IT BY DEGREES

Normally, brain temperature fluctuates by about 1.5°C (2.7°F) every day. The brain is at its minimum temperature at daybreak, and its maximum at midday. Mimicking these fluctuations could combat jetlag by reducing tiredness and tricking the brain into thinking it's a different time of day.

981 PLAN OUT TIME-ZONE PROBLEMS

Save important activities for when you have most energy – in the morning after flying west; in the evening after flying east.

982 MOVE TO PREVENT MOTION SICKNESS

On a ship or plane, move to the centre where it tends to be more stable. On a ship, go to the top deck and look out at the water to put your eyes and inner ear in sync.

983 DRINK WATER, NOT ALCOHOL

Jetlag effects are generally made worse by dehydration, caffeine and alcohol, which put stress on the body and increase fatigue.

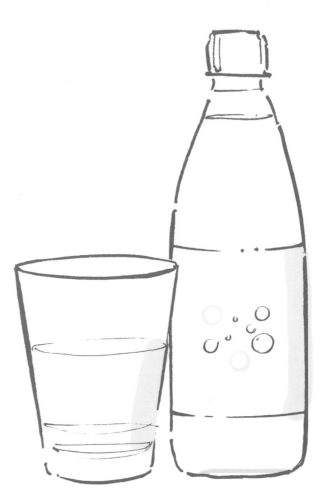

994 TREAT TRAVEL SICKNESS WITH GINGER

Ginger is a traditional herbal remedy and is available in pills, chewable ginger root and as sweets. Side effects seem to be minimal but it's always wise to check with your doctor since it has been shown to have some blood-thinning effects.

995 BE WARY OF LOCAL WATER

Local water can cause digestive upsets. Drink bottled water when abroad and be careful of fruit and salad that's washed in local water, as well as hazards like ice cubes.

treats

996 CURL UP WITH AN OLD FAVOURITE

Take ten minutes to shut yourself away with a good book or poem, or let your creative juices flow and write something yourself. Concentrating on one thing and forgetting worries will help reduce stress.

987 BOOK YOURSELF SOME SCENT TIME

Book an aromatherapy massage to relax yourself, stimulate circulation and lower stress and tension. Don't feel guilty about the time you're giving to yourself – you'll cope with life better if set aside time to enjoy the things you like to do.

988 RENT A LAUGH TO FEEL HAPPY

Give yourself a break from emotionally charged news broadcasts and mind-numbing television, or from the usual list of evening chores. Instead, rent a favourite comedy programme tape or DVD that you know will put a smile on your face.

989 BUY YOURSELF A FOODY TREAT

The next time you visit the supermarket, treat yourself to one thing that wouldn't normally be on your shopping list and, some time during the week, take time to enjoy it. Keep it healthy – such as yogurt-coated raisins, carrot cake or plain popcorn – and your treat will be guilt free!

1001 BEAT YOUR TROUBLES WITH BUBBLES

Whenever time permits, indulge in a 30-minute 'home spa' session in your own bathroom. Soak your troubles away in your favourite bubble bath; lie back, close your eyes and let pleasant thoughts flood in.

1000 SURROUND YOURSELF WITH FLOWERS

Research studies have shown that flowers provide an emotional lift. You don't need to spend a fortune to spread flowers throughout your house – buy one bouquet and split it up, putting a flower or two in several different vases.

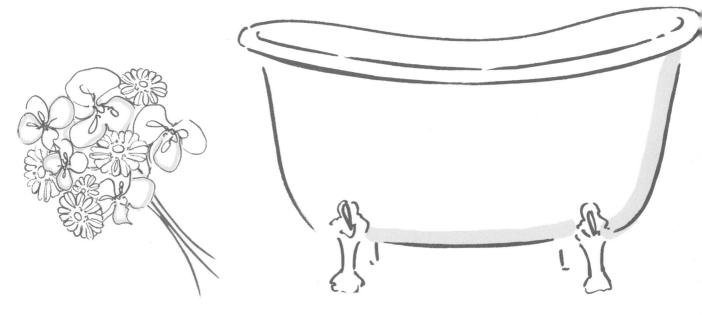